PRAISE FOR *IN THE MIRROR*

"Kaira Rouda's voice is so bright and strong she takes a difficult subject and makes it soar. Jennifer's journey through cancer and her struggle to love her husband in the face of the return of her first love, Alex, is something to cheer and rejoice in. A moving and uplifting novel about family and the struggles we all face to live every minute to the fullest."

—ANITA HUGHES, author of *Monarch Beach* and *Market Street*

"Kaira Rouda has created relatable characters you'll care deeply about. Emotionally gripping and heartachingly beautiful, *In the Mirror* will make you think about what's truly important."

—TRACEY GARVIS GRAVES, *New York Times* bestselling author

"As a reader, I was completely absorbed by *In the Mirror*. Kaira Rouda creates a main character so real and so beautifully at odds with her battle with cancer that you can't help but get completely swept up in her life-or-death journey. This is a moving story from the unique perspective of the seriously ill patient who is a mother, wife, sister, daughter, and friend, examining all those relationships with honesty and humor. *In the Mirror* is a book that will stay with you because of the questions it asks and the answers it offers."

—LIAN DOLAN, bestselling author of *Helen of Pasadena* and host of *Satellite Sisters*

"*In the Mirror* by Kaira Rouda is an emotion-packed novel about a mother facing terminal cancer. It is a nostalgic tribute to the things that really matter: family and friends. This novel is a perfect fit for readers who find a good cry to be therapeutic. The ache of the novel will be too much for many who've suffered the loss of loved ones, but for those who are in pain, who need a voice to echo what they feel, Jennifer has the feel of a friend."

—*FOREWORD REVIEWS*

PRAISE FOR KAIRA ROUDA

"I loved Kaira Rouda's book. I love its irony and its courage and humor....It's the real thing."

—JACQUELYN MITCHARD, bestselling author of *Still Summer* and *The Deep End of the Ocean*

"Reading Kaira Rouda is like getting together with one of your best friends—fun, fast, and full of great advice! *Here, Home, Hope* sparkles with humor and heart."

—CLAIRE COOK, bestselling author of *Must Love Dogs* and *Best Staged Plans*

"To be uplifted and inspired: a fabulous, inspiring, must-read for any woman who's ever thought about changing her life."

—*WOMAN'S WORLD* MAGAZINE

"Told with honest insight and humor, Rouda's novel is the story of a woman who takes charge of her life while never forgetting the people who helped make that change."

—*BOOKLIST*

"Rouda has created a lovable and perceptive heroine who navigates her struggles with honesty and awe-inspiring determination to succeed. A fun and totally satisfying read."

—AMY HATVANY, author of *Best Kept Secret*

Kaira Rouda's novels have won the Indie Excellence Book Award for Mainstream/Literary Fiction, USA Book Awards for Women's Fiction, and Honorable Mention in Writer's Digest International Book Awards.

ALSO BY KAIRA ROUDA

HERE, HOME, HOPE

ALL THE DIFFERENCE

A MOTHER'S DAY

REAL YOU INCORPORATED:
8 ESSENTIALS FOR WOMEN ENTREPRENEURS

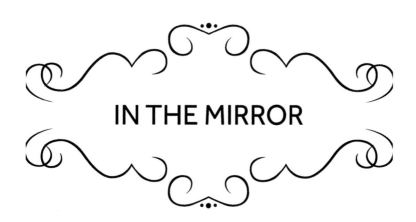

IN THE MIRROR

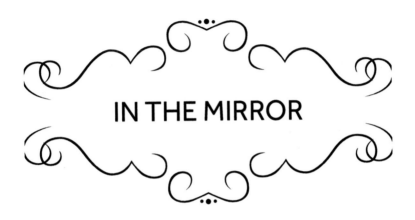

IN THE MIRROR

A NOVEL

KAIRA ROUDA

Printed in the United States of America.

ISBN: 978-0-9849151-6-3

For more about the author, visit www.KairaRouda.com.

To Trace, Avery, Shea, and Dylan

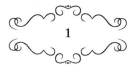

Warning: Prompt medical attention is critical for adults as well as children, even if you do not notice any symptoms.

ROLLING OVER TO GET OUT OF BED, I CAUGHT A GLIMPSE OF MYself in the mirror and cringed. My reflection said it all. Everything had changed.

I looked like death.

I blinked, moving my gaze from the mirror, and noticed the inspirational "quote of the day" calendar on my bedside table. Uplifting quote aside, it was Monday again. That meant everything in the real world, away from this place. It meant groaning about the morning and getting the kids off to school. It meant struggling to get to work on time and forcing yourself to move through the day. It meant the start of something new and fresh and undetermined. But Mondays meant nothing at Shady Valley. We lived in the "pause" world, between "play" and "stop." Suspension was the toughest part for me. And loneliness. Sure, I had visitors, but it wasn't the same as being always surrounded by people in motion. Only eighteen months ago, I'd been on fast-forward in the real world, juggling two kids and my business, struggling to stay connected to my husband, my friends.

At Shady Valley, with beige-colored day after cottage-cheese-tasting day, my pace was, well—

I had to get moving. I had a party to plan.

I supposed my longing for activity was behind my rather childish wish to throw a party for myself. At least it gave me a mission of sorts. A delineation of time beyond what the latest in a long line of cancer treatments dictated. It had been more than eighteen months of treatments, doctor's appointments, hospitalizations, and the like. I embraced the solidity of a deadline. The finality of putting a date on the calendar and knowing that at least this, my party, was something I could control.

I noticed the veins standing tall and blue and bubbly atop my pale, bony hands. I felt a swell of gratitude for the snakelike signs of life, the entry points for experimental treatments; without them, I'd be worse than on pause by now.

I pulled my favorite blue sweatshirt over my head and tugged on my matching blue sweatpants.

Moving at last, I brushed my teeth and headed next door to Ralph's. He was my best friend at Shady Valley—a special all-suite, last-ditch-effort experimental facility for the sick and dying—or at least he had been until I began planning my party. I was on his last nerve with this, but he'd welcome the company, if not the topic. He was on pause too.

My thick cotton socks helped me shuffle across my fake-wood floor, but it was slow going once I reached the grassy knoll—the leaf-green carpet that had overgrown the hallway. An institutional attempt at Eden, I supposed. On our good days, Ralph and I sometimes sneaked my son's plastic bowling set out there to compete in vicious matches. We had both been highly competitive, type-A people in the "real" world, and the suspended reality of hushed voices and tiptoeing relatives was unbearable at times.

"I've narrowed it down to three choices," I said, reaching Ralph's open door. "One: 'Please come celebrate my life on the eve of my death. RSVP immediately. I'm running out of time.'"

"Oh, honestly," Ralph said, rolling his head back onto the pillows propping him up. I knew my time in Shady Valley was only bearable because of this man, his humanizing presence. Even though we both looked like shadows of our outside, real-world selves, we carried on a relationship as if we were healthy, alive. I ignored the surgery scars on his bald, now misshapen head. He constantly told me I was beautiful. It worked for us.

"Too morbid? How about: 'Only two months left. Come see the incredible, shrinking woman. Learn diet secrets of the doomed,'" I said, hoping he'd join in.

"Jennifer, give it a rest, would you?"

"You don't have to be so testy. Do you want me to leave?" I asked, ready to retreat back to my room.

"No, come in. Let's just talk about something else, OK, beautiful?"

Ralph was lonely too. Friends from his days as the city's most promising young investment banker had turned their backs—they didn't or couldn't make time for his death. His wife, Barbara, and their three teenage kids were his only regular visitors. Some days, I felt closer to Ralph than to my own family, who seemed increasingly more absorbed in their own lives despite weekly flowers from Daddy and dutiful visits from Henry, my husband of six years. Poor Henry. It was hard to have meaningful visits at Shady Valley, with nurses and treatments and all manner of interruptions. We still held hands and kissed, but intimacy—when I was feeling up to it—was impossible.

So, there we were, Ralph and I, two near-death invalids fighting for our lives with me planning a party to celebrate that fact. It seemed perfectly reasonable, because while I knew I should be living in the moment, the future seemed a little hazy without a party to focus on.

"Seriously, I need input on my party invitations. It's got to be right before I hand it over to Mother. I value your judgment, Ralph. Is that too much to ask?"

"For God's sake, let me see them." Ralph snatched the paper out of my hand. After a moment, he handed it back to me. "The last one's the best. The others are too, well, self-pitying and stupid. And it's a good idea to keep the party manageable by scheduling groups of people. Are you sure you can't just have a funeral like the rest of us?"

I glared at him but agreed, "That's my favorite too."

Mr. & Mrs. E. David Wells
request your presence at a
celebration in honor of their daughter,
Jennifer Wells Benson.
Please see insert for your party time.
Shady Valley Center
2700 Hocking Ridge Road
RSVP to Mrs. Juliana Duncan Wells
No gifts please—donations to cancer research appreciated.

At first, I had been incredibly angry about the cancer. Hannah's birth, so joyous, also had marked the end of my life as a "normal" person. Apparently, it happened a lot. While a baby's cells multiplied, the mom's got into the act, mutating, turning on each other. Hannah was barely two weeks old when I became violently ill. My fever was 105 degrees when we arrived in the ER. I think the ER doctors suspected a retained placenta or even some sort of infectious disease, although I was so feverish I couldn't remember much from that time. All I remembered was the feeling of being cut off from my family—Henry, two-year-old Hank, and newborn Hannah—and marooned on the maternity ward, a place for mothers-to-be on bed rest until their due dates. That was hell.

My headache was so intense the curtains were drawn against the glaring sun or the streetlights at all times. I didn't look pregnant, since I wasn't anymore, so all the nurses thought my baby had died. That first shift tiptoed around me, murmuring. By the second night, one of them had posted a sign: "The baby is fine. Mother is sick." It answered their questions since I couldn't. It hurt my head too much to try.

On the third day, surgery revealed that there was no retained placenta after all. I was able to go home to my newborn and my life. With a slight fever but no answers, I escaped from the hospital and went home to a grateful Henry and a chaotic household. I was weak and tired, but everyone agreed that was to be expected. I thanked God for the millionth time for two healthy kids and my blessed, if busy, life.

Less than two weeks later, I found the lump.

Not a dramatic occurrence, really, at least not at first. I was shaving under my arm, and I happened to bump into my left breast with my hand. I felt a mass that hadn't been there before. When I pushed on the top part of my breast, closest to my underarm, it hurt. I freaked out and called for Henry.

"I'm sure it's fine," he reassured me while his eyes revealed his own fears. "We'll make an appointment to have it checked out first thing tomorrow, OK?"

Our eyes locked, and in that moment, I think we both knew.

It wasn't fine. When the radiologist at the Women's Imaging Center read the mammogram, she called my doctor right away. The spider-webby growth had spread throughout my left breast. Deadly tentacles full of cancerous cells. Surgery confirmed that the malignancy had already begun to metastasize to my lymph nodes. They moved me to the cancer floor and began treatments immediately, and that's where I'd been, in body or spirit, for more than a year.

Ralph was the one to describe them as "circle mouths": the initial reactions of family and friends expressing sympathy for our rotten luck. When the doctors finally figured out what was wrong with me, my family was the first to respond with their blank stares and circle mouths. "OOOOOO, Jennifer, we're sOOOOOO sorry." Initially, I was caught up in the angry stage of grief, enveloped by it. It ate away at my soul and left me spent, running on nothing but useless emotion. Why me? What had I done differently than anyone else I knew? Did I drink too many Diet Cokes? Eat too much McDonald's? Did I live downstream from a crop doused in pesticides? Was I a bad person? Why didn't my children deserve to grow up with a mother? Exhausted by remorse, I eventually found myself safely encased in quasi-acceptance that wrapped around me like a blanket, smothering the dreams of middle and old age and draping the vision of my children as teenagers and adults, tamping out hope I'd ever see them as such.

Hope. I knew my family thought the party was a sign that I had given up, that I was welcoming death, maybe even hastening it a bit by my bold invitation. And yet, "hope" to me was just another four-letter word without substance. I needed a reason to hang on, to continue what had become a painful and tedious daily struggle. For me, the best thing about life was the people in it. Friends, lovers, teachers, role models—they all made me the person I had become. I needed to reconnect with the living if only for a single night, to be assured my life had meant something and I was not as forgotten as I felt. No, the party was not a sign of lost hope but the opposite: a gathering of the people from my past, each a piece of some cosmic puzzle that could be configured into something whole—and healthy. Hope.

"It looks nice, Jennifer, really," Ralph said, jarring me from my reverie. "Why are your parents hosting it, though? Why not you and Henry?"

"Ah, because Juliana Duncan Wells would never forgive me if I denied her the chance to host a party. She's a professional hostess, you know."

Ralph chuckled weakly. His brown eyes were tired. I inspected his pale, thin, worn face more closely. His head, which had been shaved and cut open for multiple surgeries, was now lumpy and grooved with scars. He was an attractive man, but he had a prominent dent over his left eye, swooping to his ear. My scars were tucked away inside my cozy sweatshirt. My head was newly covered in curly blond hair. It had been straight before chemo.

I looked away. Ralph's room sported the same fake-leather chairs arranged around an imitation-wood table that mine did. I stared at green-striped walls too, and my room offered white wicker bedside tables, a fake cottage cheeriness that tried to mask the anguish of the patients who resided here. The only difference was his Naugahyde was burgundy; mine was brown.

I made my slow trek to one of the chairs and sank into it. "What's wrong today, Ralph? You seem really sad. New meds?"

"It's nothing, Jennifer, really," Ralph answered unconvincingly, clasping his thin hands together on his stomach. I noticed the incredible shrinking man had moved his platinum wedding band to his middle left finger.

I knew he was lying, but I also knew enough not to pry. Ralph Waldo Erickson—his real name, and his parents knew better—had discovered cancer when he felt a pain in his right cheek while shaving. He had a headache too. His doctor dismissed both his headache and his pain as a sinus infection when he first called. A few days later, he woke screaming in the middle of the night and was rushed to the ER, where an MRI revealed a malignant growth the size of a lemon. In the operating room, the surgeons peeled Ralph's skin to the side in order to cut out the tumor. Success—until they found more tumors. And more still, after radiation, after chemo. He was forty-five years old.

Six months earlier, he'd had a headache. Now, he had four months to live, tops.

After a few minutes of silence, he asked, with his eyes sparkling and his hands gesturing in front of him, "Did you know it's the fall harvest? I mean, all those years I drank wine—loved wine—and I didn't even take the time to learn about it. You know, learn how they make it, when they pick the grapes. God, that's sad. They're out there right now, in California, France, even Ohio, for God's sake, just outside our windows, and I never bothered to learn a thing about it. Sure, I did the touristy winery hop in Napa and Sonoma a time or two. But this is harvest season! The most beautiful time of the year, and I never bothered to be a part of it—you know?" Ralph looked up at the ceiling, clasping his hands again. I'd never noticed how long his fingers were before.

"So add it to our list, buddy, OK?" I said gently, knowing it wouldn't really help, knowing the impossibility of Ralph ever leaving Shady Valley, much less visiting Napa Valley for the harvest. "Hey, it's treatment time. I need to go back. Buzz me when you feel like it."

Ralph didn't answer, and I didn't really expect him to. We all went through depressions at Shady Valley, triggered by almost anything: harvest time or an especially beautiful orange-purple sunset. It was hard to keep your spirits up all the time. He'd be fine in a little while.

I made my way slowly back across the slick floor and padded down the thick green carpet back into my room. Promptly at four, Nurse Hadley arrived with her arsenal of vials and needles, all part of a new therapy I was determined to try.

"Well, aren't we pretty in blue," she said, as if speaking to a child.

"My veins do look stunning today," I agreed. Her eyes darted to mine. *Heck, they are nice veins,* I thought as I prepared to receive the latest experimental drug with a mixture of dread and barely detectable hope. The side effects might be hell—but still, this could be the one.

The shrill ring of the phone woke me up. Caller ID revealed it was my business partner, Jacob DuPry. I had emailed him the invitation choices, knowing he'd have an opinion since he had an opinion about everything, especially event planning.

"I'm positive you should have no more than two reception times. Period. And you know I love the idea of the party," Jacob said, exhaling loudly into the phone. I imagined him pushing his blond bangs to the right with the palm of his left hand. A signature move. "I wish dear Randolph or his partner Patrick had thought about it before they succumbed. Too late. You have more friends than they did, though. Beyond me, their death receptions would've appealed simply to the curious. But you—well, with the Loop's customers alone, you'll fill the place."

Jacob was heir apparent to our successful clothing boutique that could've been much more. Maybe Clothes the Loop would grow, still, without me. If Jacob stayed focused, he could do it.

"Life celebration, not death reception," I corrected, though I still sounded groggy from sleep. "And, just a reminder, you hated Patrick. Anyway, I just want enough time with each person—kind of like a receiving line."

I talked at the speakerphone, still lying in bed. The new miracle drug hadn't made my hair fall out, but my equilibrium was gone. I couldn't stand or shuffle to Ralph's. I had to buzz the nurses for help to the bathroom.

Thank goodness for this voice from beyond Shady Valley.

"Schedule appointments, silly. It's like we do with the trunk shows, if you want a really banal comparison," Jacob said.

"I don't," I snipped. He deserved it; he sounded distracted. "Are you paying attention?"

"Of course. I am walking to the back office right now, OK?" Jacob and I shared an office in the deepest recesses of the store, behind a door that blended into the off-white wall near the dressing rooms. We escaped to the cave whenever a customer honked us off or when we needed to console each other. "Does that make you happy? I hope so, because we are slammed and *I am walking to the back*. For you," Jacob yelled. I imagined him in his shiny black shoes, risers in the heel to make him taller. I wondered if he was a platinum- or a dirty-blond this week. "What I meant was, on the invite, tell them you'd like to spend quality time with each of them, and that you'll be up to receiving visitors during that same week. Let them decide when to visit."

"You're right," I sighed, sounding old, dead tired. Dying tired. "But where's the party in that? I want a party, Jacob."

"Have a party at the end of the week. Make it special. So you'll be happy no matter what. You might not like everyone anymore."

"Good point, but Suzanne'll be here any minute, and now I have nothing for her to typeset," I moaned, immobilized. "I'm too dizzy to use my computer."

"I'll do it. Just tell Suzanne to wait. She owes you a little time after all the printing business you've given her," Jacob said. "Don't worry, fifteen minutes. Oh no, it's Mrs. Drezner. You knew she'd walk in now. I've already dealt with Rachel White today."

"Aren't you in the back?" I asked, picturing him, the store, the activity. Missing it all, and him. Even the nosy neighbors who never bought and just snooped for gossip, like Rachel White. I'd love to hear what's going on from her about now. I didn't want to see Mrs. Drezner, though.

"Jennifer, I am in the back, but you've been away too long. Remember, I can hear her when she's at the antique store a block down the street. That loud, pinched, uptight—"

"Jacob, stop."

"I'll hide from her. Not mature, but doable. If the girls try to find me to help Mrs. Drezner, I'll sneak out the back door. Don't worry, I'll get the invite done."

And he did. He changed more than I thought he should, but I liked it. Suzanne, the busybody owner of the local print shop, who for some reason spoke with a hint of a Southern accent, didn't.

"You'd think from reading this Henry wasn't in the picture or somethin', honey," she said, scanning the email on my screen. I had to give her credit: she had tried to sit still until the email came in. I'd watched as she uncomfortably folded her rounded body into one of my brown square chairs. The sun streaked in over her shoulder, so I couldn't see her face, but I guessed it registered impatience. I was too dizzy to care.

"Why? Because Mother's the RSVP? She wants to do it," I said. As the wife of the local king of burgers, she had presided over many a restaurant opening in Daddy's chain.

"How about, 'Please Join Henry Benson in celebrating the life of…'" Suzanne suggested. I could tell she was pacing—her voice kept coming from different places in the room—but I didn't open my eyes.

"Fine," I said.

"I'll typeset both versions. Send it to you. Show it to your mom, Henry, whoever. Then call and we'll go with whatever you want, honey. OK? I've gotta go, gotta get back to the city."

"Sure, I know how it is," I said. I did. Suzanne's hatred of what Shady Valley represented exuded from her every word and movement.

It was an unimaginable place for her, a place of fixed positions and waiting, yet here I was.

"OK, glad to see you, Jennifer. Really. You look great. Whatever they're doing must be really working. You'll be outta here in no time. I'll email you, OK? Great. See ya soon," Suzanne said. The tap-tap of her high heels on my fake-wood floor picked up speed and ended before the word "great." The last words were from the hall. She was gone.

Not that I was really hearing her—certainly not caring. I pushed my nurse call button.

"Yes, Jennifer?"

I hated to call them unless it was an emergency. I knew they kept track of who pushed the button and when. Too many times and they got revenge: no response, or at the very least, a really slow response. In the middle of the night, it better be death knocking on your door if you buzzed them.

"Sorry to bother you, but this latest treatment is, well, I'm still dizzy, and I think I'm getting worse." I sounded so helpless. I hated that, but I hated the way the room was pitching and swaying more.

"We'll call your doctor, Jennifer, and see what he recommends."

Probably what he'd recommend would be to stop looking for a miracle, stop looking for a future. We'd exhausted his supply of hope. "Please, doctor, money's no object." Henry pushing, then my mother, and Henry again. "We're doing all we can. All I know to do," Dr. Chris, my exhausted oncologist, would tell them.

"Do more, doctor," my mother said, like she could simply charge it on her platinum American Express card. "Whatever you can find, you should try." Though she'd never smoked, she had a breathy, B-movie actress voice. She had kissed Elvis on screen once. She used her "kissing Elvis look"—straight in the eyes—while talking with Dr. Chris. He was forced to look away.

And behind it all, I guess, I pushed the hardest. After all, I had the most to lose.

My son, Hank, believed lightning was God taking pictures, and when I went to heaven, he'd know I was taking lots of pictures of him when the storms came. Death was pretty clear-cut for him, really. Poof, I'd be gone, up to heaven. Taking flash photos. At first, I hadn't wanted to tell him that Mommy might not get better. I wanted to hold him and promise him everything would be all right and that I would be the strong, happy mommy I hoped he could still remember from his toddlerhood. But after six months of hospital visits and guilty silence whenever he entered the room, he knew "Mommy's sick" didn't quite cover it. He was one smart cookie, my Hank. Henry and I decided to level with him when I moved to Shady Valley, and he absorbed the possibility of my demise with the heartbreaking practicality of a three-year-old. I would still be his mommy, just in the clouds, taking photos.

Tears threatened to overtake me whenever I thought too much about the kids. Fifteen months without a mother at home. Baby Hannah had only known what it was like to have me rock her to sleep or tuck her in at night in her crib a few blessed times, in between hospital stays and when I wasn't too ill at home. Paige was a wonderful nanny, a godsend really, but she wasn't me.

Anger mixed with sadness choked me. I wanted to brush my teeth, but I couldn't get up. I felt helplessness overwhelm me. This living in the moment thing was hell. Where was Henry? He was supposed to be coming for our "date night," as we lamely called them. What time was it anyway?

There was a time when he couldn't keep his hands off of me, my Henry. Our first year of marriage was now something of a dream. Making love in the morning before work; some days, meeting at our condo at noon for more. Evenings were filled with workouts at the gym, dinners out, and more sweet, slow lovemaking. Beyond work, no outside distractions, no kiddos yet, no responsibilities except to discover each other.

"I've never been this happy," he whispered to me as we cuddled in bed the evening of our first anniversary. It was a beautiful, starry night, and we had shared a candlelit dinner on our patio.

"Because I've finally learned how to cook?" I teased, looking up into his sparkling blue eyes. To say I hadn't really mastered any meal would be an understatement. That evening I'd created gaz-pacho from scratch. I didn't realize, though, that garlic cloves are pieces of garlic bulbs. I'd added eight bulbs. We both took our first bites—and spit them out at the same time.

"Yes, your cooking is the reason, clearly," Henry answered, chuck-ling as he rolled over on top of me. "What you lack in the kitchen you more than make up for in the bedroom. Happy anniversary, love of my life," he added before we made love again.

"Hi, honey. Weather Channel again?" Henry said when he walked in my door. I had wanted to look good, a little attractive or at least not smelly, when he arrived, but the dizziness had kept me from getting ready. I pulled the sheet up over my face and struggled to throw off my dark mood. I didn't want to waste what little time we shared these days with pointless self-pity.

"Did you know storms turn to the right after dark? I just heard that," I said through the sheet. I could see Henry through the thin fabric—the handsome man who used to want to touch me all over. Now we discussed the weather.

Henry's cleft chin nodded in my direction. "The nurses said you had a tough day. They're still waiting for Dr. Chris to figure out something to counteract the dizziness. They'll figure it out. Now pull the covers down. You know I think you look fine just how you are. I brought your favorite pasta, and a work problem for you to help me with, so get that sheet off your face and give me a kiss."

I pulled the sheet down slowly as Henry smiled, then bent over and kissed my forehead. More brotherly than affectionate, but at least he still cared enough to kiss me. It wasn't the passionate, intense kiss of our life before kids, nor was it the amazed, team-spirited kiss we used to share when we were both exhausted new parents and Hank was finally asleep. No, these kisses were those of a friend, a caring companion, a long-lost uncle. I don't know where the old kisses went, or how, if ever, to get them back.

Tonight I was dizzy, but sometimes on our date nights, I had felt OK. Shady Valley wasn't a place conducive to making love, of course, but still. Lately, he had seemed more and more distracted, and I struggled to find topics to hold his interest. New meds and side effects only took us so far. In the old days, he had shared every detail of his day with me and often asked my advice about work issues. He was passionate about life, about our relationship and me. He'd swoop in from work and grab me in a tight hug and lingering kiss. He loved his job and was determined to be the best, and I loved that about him. He still made an effort to share bits and pieces of his life with me, but I couldn't shake the sensation that he was just going through the motions for my sake.

"You would not believe what an idiot Bill Jackson is," I remember him complaining once as he swept into our condo and grabbed me in a bear hug. I'd been rummaging through our refrigerator, trying to decide if I should attempt a meal. After a big kiss, he explained his boss's latest rainmaker scheme for the law firm, which involved Henry joining the board of almost every nonprofit in town.

"But honey, it does seem like a good way to get your name out there—and your firm's name out there," I answered. I poured him a glass of Chianti and carried it to him where he sat fuming in his favorite chair. Our condo was furnished in a just-starting-out manner: one gray leather couch, one coffee table, one gray leather side chair. We had both told our parents we didn't want help with furniture, so we were working and acquiring things slowly. His favorite chair was really our only chair.

"That's not the point. You shouldn't join boards of charities unless you believe in them. And I want to specialize in business start-ups," he said.

"Well, a lot of nonprofits are run like small businesses," I offered. "I'll help you find a couple that would be a good fit. Maybe even a small-business incubator/funding group."

"I love you, Jenn," Henry said, and I climbed on his lap. "Once I'm here with you, nothing else matters."

Now, I pulled my sheet back over my head. *What matters now?* I wondered. In high school, Henry's prowess on the football field had made him quite the heartthrob. At thirty-five, his sandy-blond hair was definitely thinning, but he still had the broad shoulders and air of confidence that turned heads in a crowd. I loved that—as long as I was standing beside him. *But now, he's out in the real world, turning heads, making deals, and I'm here.*

Together, we had made a picture-perfect pair. In the early years of our marriage, we were always in the social pages, smiling, successful, in love. Henry came from a much more demonstrative family than mine, and he was constantly holding my hand, hugging and kissing me in public. When we first started dating, I blushed constantly, unaccustomed to the overt attention and the pulsing sexual tension underlying each of our dates. Our relationship started out magnetic and intense—and it was obvious to those around us. During our first date, over lunch, the air pulsed around us. When our fingers accidentally touched as he passed me the bread, I had felt the touch everywhere on my body. And wanted more. A few months later, my friend Maddie Wilson, the city's gossip columnist, described us as the couple "most in need of a cold shower or a quick exit from every fund-raiser" in her annual awards. Of course, I had blushed and Henry had laughed.

I wondered if he ever felt as lonely as I did. He had to. Even though that initial head-over-heels attraction had waned somewhat with the arrival of kids and a busy life, we still had had a vibrant sex life. Before now. Did his healthy body crave the warmth and companionship of someone equally strong and vibrant? Every inch of me had been poked and prodded, radiated, and shot with chemicals. The doctors warned us that sexual intercourse would be tough during some treatments, with vaginal dryness, early menopause, and other physical…blessings, as the social worker encouraged me to consider them. But they said we should try to maintain intimacy. Touching. Holding hands. As much as I could tolerate, as much as Henry and I could naturally feel in this unnatural state, this artificial place. Until today, and until these new meds, I'd felt as if we could try to have sex. But with the room swooping, I felt lucky being able to communicate.

I looked up at Henry. *How does he see me now? As a wife? As a lover?* At six feet three, Henry exuded vitality, while I seemed to be shrinking by the day. Would he notice if I disappeared entirely? Or would he be relieved it was over at last?

"Pull the sheet down honey," Henry said. "Your mother said Alex Thomas is back in town. Did you know that?"

Alex Thomas…

I kept the sheet over my face so Henry couldn't see me blush. My ex-boyfriend, here. In town. My past, back in my present.

And something in me wanted to see him.

2

Warning: Keep this and all drugs out of the reach of children.

ALEXANDER CALDWELL THOMAS. HIS FAMILY WAS WELL KNOWN in town because his parents owned a major furniture store, but that wasn't why I liked him, of course. He was gorgeous and kind—and he was my first boyfriend. Our first private kiss was in tenth grade, after he drove me home from a party. Our first public kiss was by the school bicycle stands the next Monday. It was lunchtime, and I was in the quad with a group of my friends. He walked over to where I was standing and asked if he could talk to me. My friends—who knew about my new crush—laughed as I blushed and followed him to a corner by the bike stands.

"I had a great time with you Saturday night," Alex said. His soft brown eyes, dark hair, and white teeth, the lines of his chin and cheeks were the same as in my dreams since Saturday night.

"Me too," I said, knowing I was blushing and glad I had dressed just for him in my best jeans and a baby-blue T-shirt I knew fit well.

"You have beautiful eyes," he said and brushed my hair from my face while leaning in for a kiss. On the lips. A tender, nectarine-in-the-sun kiss. My first public kiss, my second kiss ever.

"Can we see each other tonight, maybe?" Alex asked.

"Yes." I felt my face flush again. I would've gone anywhere, done anything with Alex back then.

And for a while, we were inseparable. We talked on the telephone for hours. Ate lunch together. Held hands at the movies. On the weekends, we'd hang out with other couples. We went to homecoming that fall. The furniture heir and the burger princess, a perfect couple. Healthy, young, full of life and possibilities.

In the same town as that dance but what felt like millions of miles from it, I smelled Mother's approach—Chanel No. 5, thick, long lasting, and rich—before she reached the end of the green-carpeted hallway and knocked on my partially opened door. It was too late to sneak into the bathroom, feigning sickness. Usually, that worked. She couldn't disguise her hatred for people with colds or the flu; throwing up killed her.

When she entered the room, my mother, Juliana stared at me. Fortunately, my room had stopped spinning, so I was able to smile back. Her poofy gray hair—just done, because it seemed she was always having it done—was as perfect as her face, graced by the skill of the best plastic surgeons in Florida three times so far. Her eyes sparkled with complements from her diamond choker.

Suddenly, I wanted Hannah to have that choker. Juliana couldn't give my sister all of it. There was so much, too much. "Hi, Mother. Can Hannah have that choker someday?" I blurted.

"Are you all right, dear?" Juliana asked, not moving closer, simply hovering as she pasted concern onto her perfect face. I remembered that, as a baby, Hank had burst into tears whenever my mother spoke. He hated her voice.

No, Mother, I'm dying, I almost said, but I needed Hannah to have that necklace. "I'm fine, Mother, really. I just love that necklace."

"You always have, dear. You know it's the one Donald gave me, just before I said yes to your father," she answered, perched on the edge of one of my Naugahyde chairs, reminding me that she was quite the catch back in the day with suitors seeming to drop jewelry on her daily. She never settled in anywhere. "Since you were a little girl, you loved this necklace," she said thoughtfully, stroking it. "Yes, that would be nice. For Hannah. I'll make sure she has it, dear. How's that?"

"That's nice. Thank you, Mother. So what are you doing today?" I asked, attempting a shift in our typical idle banter.

"I am going to the Labor Day Arts Festival, so I don't have much time," she answered, flashing one of her square smiles, her fake smile, while she glanced at her Cartier watch.

"Of course." I smiled back. Fortunately, I had inherited my dad's smile shape—an orange-slice smile. Juliana and my sister, Julie, smiled squares. You could never tell if a square smile was sincere. At least I couldn't.

"Julie wants to visit this week, if that would be all right with you," Mother said.

"Is she in town again?" I asked, feeling a cartoon anvil drop onto my chest at the mention of her name. It wasn't a cartoon, though. It was Julie. My sister.

"Yes, she is. But not with Mark—well, you know. She and the girls decided it would be fun to visit, and of course your father and I love having them at the house, so we said come and stay for as long as you like. So, there," Juliana reported, beginning to pace in her pageant walk. It signified her need to not discuss Julie with me, her need to leave and be at an arts festival. I noticed her shoes were the same sky blue as her suit. She could've been the mother of the bride again.

"How long have they been in town, Mother?" I realized this was the reason Juliana didn't visit last week.

"Just a few days, dear. So can I tell her that she can come for a visit, then? Maybe tomorrow? She's going to the arts festival with me, and I really need to scoot for today."

"Sure, scoot along. I'm not going anywhere. Tell Julie whenever."

As usual, Mother simply pretended I hadn't sounded sarcastic. That was the Juliana way of handling most of life's unpleasant situations. Ignore them and they will disappear. I sensed she resented my cancer in part because it couldn't be ignored.

"I'll have her call first," she said. "Would you like a new painting for over there?" she asked, pointing a perfectly manicured fire-engine-red fingernail at the green-striped wall in front of her, near the door. "I'll look for one, dear. I think that would be good," she added, walking up closer to the wall and pivoting, in her sky-blue, beauty-queen way. "Your friend Kelly just started a home staging company. Maybe I'll have her come in here and really spruce this place up. What do you think?"

"Thanks for the offer, but I'm not planning on staying here that much longer. I do appreciate you coming, Mother," I said, and I meant it. At least she had tried.

The most awkward part of our visit occurred, as it always did, at the end. Juliana hated physical contact, at least with other women. Especially sick women. I watched as she walked slowly to my bedside. Gingerly, she rested her hand on my shoulder, then bent and placed an overly moist kiss on my cheek.

"I do think you look better today. Yes, you are getting better," Mother said, hustling out of the room.

"Tell Daddy I'm expecting a visit," I yelled. I waited until she was almost gone, tapping down the dark green carpet before I tossed out my daddy line. I was Daddy's girl; she and I both knew it. Why did I rub it in? Because I needed him, that's why. She had Julie. I needed to know I still had Daddy on my side in our Wells version of *Family Feud*.

The rest of the morning passed in a blur of routine tests and monitoring everything. Fortunately no more drugs today. I thought about Ralph. I hadn't seen him since the day before. He had looked worried, then, not sad. Worried. He'd been told he'd die soon, so what was left to worry about?

After lunch—a despicable arrangement of bland unidentifiable foodstuff that I pushed around and made miniature sand castles with—I was startled out of my food-play reverie when Ralph leaned in my doorway with a lost-puppy grin. "So did you just decide to never come back for a visit?" It was good to see him, of course. It was good to stop thinking.

"Well, you were a grump yesterday, so I decided to play hard to get," I answered, from my throne—what I sometimes called my bed. Ralph moved well with his walker. I wondered if I'd need one of those soon. "Has Barbara come, by the way? I haven't seen her for a couple of days."

Ralph deflated in front of my eyes. What had I done by asking? It wasn't my business, interfering in their terminal-illness marriage dance. Every couple had to handle this differently, with unique rhythm.

"She said she needed a break, and she just couldn't come here this week. That her life was falling apart and that she couldn't handle it, you know, handle me dying," Ralph said, choking on the words, trying not to cry even as his shoulders sagged. I was relieved he made it to the cocktail table and maneuvered his walker so that he was able to drop into the closest brown chair. "I guess she figures since she has all the time in the world, it's OK. Maybe she's given all she can."

My heart ached for Ralph, and Barbara too. I supposed Barbara had given it all her heart, and all her hope, to get their life back to the way it was BC, before cancer. Maybe she couldn't do it anymore. *How long will Henry hold out?* I wondered.

"This is hard. I know you know," Ralph continued. "It'd probably be easier if I'd just been hit by a car. Easier on Barb and the kids. Shit. I'm sorry to bother you with this."

This. Our matching, sterile rooms. Our matching, desolate fates. He wasn't bothering me—he was showing me what I didn't want to have happen, what couldn't happen. I needed him to get through this, for his marriage and for mine.

"Ralph, you're my best friend these days. You know I'm here for you. See, I'm creeping over as we speak," I said. And I was. When I got to his side at last, I stooped and hugged him gently around the neck.

"God, you're beautiful!" He turned and kissed me firmly on the lips.

"Ralph!" I said, shocked, pushing back from him. I hadn't kissed another man since I started dating Henry, and before that, since I was with my longtime boyfriend Alex. I loved Ralph like a brother, not a lover.

Surprisingly, though, the kiss had felt nice. His kiss stirred something deep inside, something I thought was gone.

"Sorry, Jennifer. Please forgive me. I'm just lonely, I guess. I've dreamed of doing that, you know. Except in my dreams we're both healthy and we're outside, in a vineyard, I think. Anyway, I'm sorry. Still my best friend?"

"Sure." I stood there, feeling weak in the knees, not knowing where to sit. I decided I would insult him if I shuffled back to the throne, so I parked in the other chair. "Boy, you're a mess. But a good kisser. Do you know I haven't kissed anybody but Henry on the lips since I was married? Six years of no lips on anybody else."

"Sorry," Ralph said again, looking down at his hands.

"It's OK. I'm flattered, actually. It's nice to feel like I'm attractive to somebody—it makes me feel alive. Kind of counteracts that whole body-trying-to-kill-itself thing," I said. "We are still lovable, even though we are different, look different." It had felt nice, but only because it wouldn't happen again, and we both knew it. I thought for a moment.

"Do you ever dream of old girlfriends when you and Barbara get in a fight? Like now, do you think you're fantasizing about me to block her or get even in your mind or something?" I asked.

"Maybe," he said, shifting in his chair, clearly uncomfortable with our talk, but a smile was sneaking onto his face. "I told you I've been dreaming about you. I guess Barb's the reason, or our lack of relationship is the reason. And God, I'm lonely. And, well, you are gorgeous, Jenn—inside and out."

"Thanks, Ralph, so are you," I said. "I remember I used to dream about Alex, my high school boyfriend, whenever Henry and I would fight. It was weird. Still, I think about what my life would've been like if I'd married him instead of Henry. It is a fascinating thing, the mind. That's why we hang on to hope. And the future. Mind over body, whatever it takes, including the healing power of touch," I added, reaching over to hold his hand. I didn't mention I'd had my own vivid dream of Alex a few nights earlier. We sat close, enjoying a bonfire on a farm an hour's drive away from town. We were so young, so in love. His dark eyes sparkled in the glow of the fire. His lips, perfect and red. His dark thick hair falling carelessly over his right eye. Our lives were full of possibility, carefree and sexy. I shook my head, trying to eliminate those thoughts of the past, no matter how stimulating. Ralph needed me now.

"You need to believe that the woman you love just needs a respite. That she is tired and grumpy, and that's all," I said, trying to focus on Ralph and not Alex. "Because I've watched her care for you, Ralph, and she loves you so much. Almost as much as you love her."

Tears streamed down his cheeks as I rose to embrace him again, minus the kiss. "Do you really think she still loves me, Jenn? I'm pretty sure I don't love myself right now."

"Of course she does," I answered but wasn't sure. I wasn't sure about anything these days. Who could know what was in someone else's heart? I had loved Alex before Henry. When Henry came along, I loved him enough to marry him, even though Alex had asked me repeatedly through college. Henry loved the me he had met, but did he love me now? Like this? Maybe Ralph was right. We'd lost the ability to love ourselves.

I patted his shoulder and said, "I'm going to get ready for later. You can stay here." I made my way, slowly, into the bathroom. I could hear him crying as I shut the door.

Henry and the kids were coming tonight, and I needed lots of time to get ready, since during Henry's last visit, I hadn't been able to move. I had a nifty chair in the bathroom, and another little sitting spot in the shower, so I could primp and not wear myself out. Sometimes I was more like my mother than I liked to admit, even to myself. After I finished my makeup, I decided Ralph needed a rousing game of Scrabble to distract him. We were fierce Scrabble opponents.

But when I emerged from the bathroom, dressed in a stunning purple sweat suit emboldened with a white heart on the top—a look that screamed health and happiness and made it impossible to be anything but cheerful—I found Suzanne and Ralph reviewing party invitations. Ralph was all smiles, and Suzanne was actually flirting.

"I see you two have met," I said as Suzanne jumped up from the brown chair to let me sit.

"I think you're really going to love them, Jennifer. Ralph here has already picked out his favorite," Suzanne said, smiling at Ralph. *He is cute but married,* I thought at her, *and dying, for heaven's sake.*

"Oh good, because it's hard for me to make a decision without Ralph," I said sarcastically. Was I jealous? "I'm kidding. I appreciate your advice. Both of you."

> *Please join*
> *Henry, Jennifer, Hank, and Hannah Benson*
> *in a celebration of Jennifer's life*
> *the week of September 10.*
> *Appointments will be accepted for Monday, Wednesday, and Friday*
> *to ensure our quality time together.*
> *Please RSVP with your intentions to Jennifer's mother,*
> *Juliana Duncan Wells, by September 1.*
> *In lieu of gifts, please donate to the breast cancer charity of your choice.*

"I like it, Suzanne." I really did. "With Henry, Hank, and Hannah included. Great."

"I'll drop off a copy for your mother, if you'd like," Suzanne offered. "If your mom likes it, we'll get the engraving plates tomorrow, and I'd guess you could have them the first of next week. You know, it does sound like a truly wonderful party, Jennifer," Suzanne said. Was she batting her eyes at Ralph? Too bad she wouldn't be invited. Neither would Ralph, if he didn't get his sex drive under control.

"Sounds good, Suzanne. Don't you need to get back to the city? Busy-busy and all?" I asked. I *was* jealous.

"You know, you're right, honey. So nice to meet you, Ralph. I hope I'll see you the next time I'm here," she said, shaking his hand again while gathering up her sample book. "I'll let you know if your mother has any problems with the invite, Jennifer."

I grumpily pulled out the Scrabble board, planning to beat Ralph in revenge. I was good with words; I won my sixth-grade spelling bee.

I hoped Barbara surfaced soon, or the stud muffin could become dangerous. Ralph flirted during our entire game, spelling sexual innuendos whenever he could. I ended up killing him. He said the only reason I beat him was because he was tired. *Ha.* The real reason was his raging hormones. Scrabble was too wholesome to handle a board full of obscenities.

While we were playing—and flirting—our way through Scrabble, I thought about the long weekends in college when Alex and I would play board games. As I smiled at Ralph, I saw Alex's eyes. I shook my head and concentrated on my remaining three letters: *C A T.* Rearranged, they were Alex Caldwell Thomas's initials. A surge of energy pulsed through me at the realization, as did the image of a particularly romantic kiss we shared at a restaurant on the left bank in Paris. We'd been drinking at a booth in the back, sharing a heaping bowl of mussels. The restaurant was crowded, dark, and smoky when he grabbed my ponytail and pulled me in for a forceful, deep kiss. Amazing.

I needed help. This wasn't healthy. I was a happily married woman with two children. "Ralph, I'm stuck—you win," I said, lying and tossing my remaining letters into the black bag. "Pastor Barker will be here any minute, and he cannot see this board of sin," I added.

"You are right about that, Jenn," Ralph said as we quickly cleaned up. He began to make his way out of my room, then turned and said, "I know I apologized earlier, for the kiss. But it was one of the best things that happened to me here in this place, as are you. So I'm not really sorry." And he was out the door.

Pastor Paul Barker was scheduled to come for our weekly devotional. I was relieved, as usual, that he couldn't read my mind, or he might've thought our sessions weren't worth it. I had always believed in grace. And forgiveness. And heaven. Had I thought about them a lot before? No, probably like a lot of people, I thought about God mostly when I needed help in life—when troubles came my way.

Now, I wanted desperately to believe but found I had far too many questions to rely on faith alone. My lack of conviction scared me as much as it worried the good Pastor Barker. When I turned nine, my grandmother gave me a necklace with a tiny seed enclosed in a bottle suspended from a delicate silver chain. A mustard seed. The idea was to inspire me to move mountains, of course, but I lost it pretty much right away. Pastor Barker had assured me, when I only half-jokingly confessed this small mistake with what I suspected was major symbolism, that God did not hold that against me. But I had more realistic concerns, which Pastor Barker did want to help me with. And the fact I had been kissed by another man, dreamed about my old boyfriend, and played X-rated Scrabble only added to my troubles.

I heard a quiet knock. "Jennifer, may I come in?" Pastor Barker said, standing just outside my door. Polite—he was so polite.

"Please do," I called. I felt pretty good, since the dizziness had subsided early this morning after whatever concoction they'd tried. I decided to sit in one of my squeaky vinyl chairs for our talk. I dangled my legs over the edge of the bed. Fine, good. Slipping down, my legs held, and I shuffled—really more of a slow walk. Pastor Barker helped me settle into my chair before sitting in the ugly matching one, table between us. He was tall, maybe six feet four, and hopelessly tried to find a way to sit comfortably.

As I watched Pastor Barker in the chair, I imagined the biggest sea lion trying to make room on the rock, wiggling back and forth until all the other sea lions scooched over. Too bad armrests weren't sea lions.

"Let's talk about life's contradictions today, OK?" I suggested, trying to erase the sea lion image and get right down to business. I needed some answers today.

"In what regard, Jennifer?" he asked. His eyes were gray and kind.

"Life isn't fair, really. I mean, why does God make it so tempting to want to live when heaven is supposedly so much better? He gave me a husband, beautiful children, a home, loving friends, but now he's taking them all away. That's what I don't understand," I said.

"But don't you see? God heaped on the blessings for your life, condensed them, in a sense, so you've lived a very full life, even if it may be a shortened one," Pastor Barker answered, reaching for my hand for emphasis. "You are going to a better place, to plan a place in your new home for Henry and the children, when it's their time. They will grow up knowing they have a special angel in heaven watching over them."

I'd heard it before, I thought, breaking eye contact and swinging my right foot along the floor. Yeah, in other words, I'd be taking a lot of pictures. "I'd rather be taking them for swimming lessons," I said. I needed him to tell me more, give me more. He was hard to stay mad at, though.

"Would you? I mean, if God gave you back all the time in the world, now, today, would you do what you had always done? Live the same life?"

Ah, a perfect pastor problem. I stopped swinging my leg, but I'd thought this one through. "No, of course not. I'd sell the store to Jacob. I'd spend more time with the kids. I'd take those classes and get my MBA like I always wanted, and I'd travel more with Henry instead of always putting it off, and…" Tears choked off my words, and I just squeaked, "I'm sorry."

"Tears are fine, Jennifer. I'm accustomed to them," Pastor Barker said, standing to reach for a box of tissues. "This isn't meant to be torturous. Whatever time God gives us on this earth, we humans fill it up. Mostly with meaningless, day-to-day activities. That is, after all, the process we call living. We forget to cherish, celebrate every moment as the blessing it is. We live for the future, the next thing. Many people don't have a final warning, a time before death: a transition period to prepare themselves and their families for their deaths. When I counsel parents who lose children suddenly or children who lose parents or spouses who lose spouses, they always wish they had a chance to say good-bye. Always."

"But what does the person who died wish?" I asked, sniffing.

"Eternal life, Jennifer," he answered.

"No, really, I bet what they want was that drunk driver not to murder them, or not to drown in the lake, or whatever. They wanted to live, presumably—even people who commit suicide want to live," I said. I knew the point he was trying to make, but I just didn't think he got it. Without talking to somebody who was dead, he'd never have the answers I needed, no matter how much I tried to believe. No matter how much I needed to believe.

"What about Henry? Our relationship? It's like we're not even married anymore. I'm more of a child he has to visit and take care of," I said, blowing my nose into the tissue. "I know the for-better-and-worse stuff, but this—I am no longer what he signed up for."

"Don't be ridiculous. Henry loves you. Together you will fight this and, God willing, come through together. Stronger."

I understood, but I wasn't convinced. Kids challenge a relationship. A move to another city challenges a relationship. Unemployment, financial worries, infidelity—all of those life hurdles challenge a marriage. Death, the fact that it may arrive sooner than expected, shakes the foundation of everything.

"But I don't think he loves me the same way anymore. Look at me. Would you want to make love to me?" I asked. Realizing I'd made Pastor Barker blush, I added: "What I mean is, the romance is gone."

"Jennifer, romantic love wanes in every couple. There are times when we are each other's companions, each other's best friends, and times when we are each other's passionate lovers. That is the reality of long-term, committed relationships. It is also a reality that no one lives forever," Pastor Barker said. "Eventually, most of us receive a terminal diagnosis, and we're lucky if our partner stands with us in our fight, like Henry is for you. We all go on to a better place. No suffering. No cancer treatments. No more exhaustion." He leaned forward so his face perched very close to mine. I slumped lower in the chair. "Shall we pray?" he asked, placing his hand on my hand.

"Sure," I said. That was his sign he was finished with me for this week. I bowed my head as he led us in prayer. I listened while he blessed Hannah and Hank and Henry, but my thoughts drifted again. To tell the truth, Pastor Barker's religion seemed too fatalistic. I mean, he focused on the afterlife while I still had hope for more of this life. I prayed for a cure while he prayed for a soft spot in heaven for me. *What if his prayers negate mine?* I thought in panic. *What if his were stronger because he didn't lose his mustard seed?*

Pastor Barker expected me to accept my fate with grace, but I wanted a miracle, just like in the Bible: blindness cured, leprosy healed, death banished. "Daughter, your faith has made you well"—it could happen, couldn't it?

"Amen," Pastor Barker said, interrupting my reverie.

"Amen," I answered, looking up into his sad, gray eyes. He was a sailor. Loved to be on the water. I knew he'd love to be there instead of with me.

"Shall I come by next Tuesday, Jennifer?"

"Of course, I look forward to our time together," I said. And then, feeling guilty, I added, "You know, I'm planning a party, and I'd love for you to come. I'm hoping to get the invitations in the mail by Friday."

"A party? Well, of course, we'd love to come. Shall I help you back to your bed?" polite Pastor Barker asked.

"Yes, thank you. Aren't you impressed I sat with you this entire time? I think I'm getting better. Maybe this new experimental drug is working. Clobbering those cancer cells. I'm feeling a little of my old spunk coming back," I said, shuffling my socks over the fake-wood floor as his strong hand held me under my left armpit. Maybe he thought my red sweatpants and top were too flashy.

"I'd love to see that spunk back. We all would. We'll keep you in our prayers this week," he said.

"*Healing* prayers. Right, Pastor Barker?" I couldn't stop myself from asking.

"Of course, Jennifer. Of course," Pastor Barker answered sadly. I had to wonder.

After pulling my blanket up over me, Pastor Barker turned and walked out the door and back to the real world of births and baptisms; of marriages, affairs, and divorces; and of sicknesses and nonquestioning sudden death. As for me, I'd decided that even if I didn't look like it on the outside, I was starting to feel like my old self on the inside. And that was what I'd be holding on to. I considered turning on my laptop, even, and checking some long-neglected emails. Maybe I'd be well enough to go on a buying trip this fall with Jacob, or maybe this spring. Maybe Henry and I could go on a date? I could get my sexy back, I knew I could. But first, I'd close my eyes.

I slept for a long time after Pastor Barker left. The talk had been draining, as they often were. The peace I searched for every time he appeared was short-lived, but my inward resolve felt stronger. I felt stronger. When Hadley brought my afternoon snack tray, I told her I wasn't hungry. That resulted in vicious nonverbal disapproval, but I didn't care.

Suddenly, I heard laughter working its magic, floating down the green hall and rushing like a gurgling waterfall into my room. My heart swelled. Hank was the kind of kid everybody wanted to take home: he was warm, bubbly, and had curly blond hair and soft, fair skin. He loved to laugh, and he loved to cuddle. If I tickled him, his laugh turned deeper and rhythmic, sounding exactly like Woody Woodpecker's. He bounded into my room wearing his new hiking boots with plastic bugs imbedded in the clear plastic soles.

"Look at my bug boots, Mommy," he said, running over to my bed and trying to hoist his little foot up high enough for me to see the bottom.

"Cool, champ, I love 'em. Can you climb up here with me?"

"Sure, Mommy. How you doin' today?" Hank asked, carrying the step stool over to the bed. He also carried it into my bathroom to go "tinkle" when he needed to. He was very self-sufficient, my little man. As he snuggled next to me, my heart swelled with pride and love. And longing. I longed to be there for him.

Paige waddled in, her legs straddling a beaming Hannah, whose tiny hands grasped each of Paige's as she perfected her baby gait. She had taken her first steps about a month earlier—three months later than Hank, who walked at ten months.

"Hi, baby girl!" I said as she rounded the corner. She had an orange-slice smile, which was almost filled in with teeth. In greeting, she screeched. I loved that—a gleeful sound almost as captivating as Hank's giggle.

"I get Mommy first, Hann-baby," Hank said angrily, looking down from the bed at his little sister.

"Don't worry, Hank. You can cuddle me as long as you'd like," I said as he stretched out his little body on top of mine, positioning his head just under my chin, bug boots digging into my thigh.

"Do you want me to take those off?" Paige asked, pointing at the boots.

"No, that's OK. Hank's very proud of them. I am too," I said, rubbing his head.

Hank was born about a year after I started my business with Jacob. Clothes the Loop was doing great, and Henry and I were ready to begin a family. We'd been married almost two years. As luck would have it—and we felt truly lucky back then—I got pregnant on the first try. No birth control pills and *bam*, knocked up.

Hank, tired of cuddling, pushed off of me and angled his bug boots toward the stool. Paige swooped and carried him, boots and all, to the toy chest in the corner of my room. After getting him settled in, she brought me Hannah—who didn't want to be held.

"Eehhhhhhhhh," she screeched, arching her tiny back in protest. *Why didn't she know I needed to hold her? Why couldn't she cuddle?* I wondered. Because she was on the verge of toddlerhood. I wanted her to be independent. She'd need to be, if her mom didn't make it.

"That's OK, Paige. Maybe Henry'll bring her back later tonight, before bed. Then she'll want to snuggle," I said, grinning but avoiding looking at Paige. I didn't want her to see the tears about to overrun my eyelashes.

"We bought all the supplies for preschool today. And, of course, Hank got to pick out his new school shoes. I think he's really looking forward to it," Paige said, helping keep my tears away with chatter. "I met the teachers yesterday. They said to call if you have questions. I brought all the handouts. They're in with the rest of your mail."

"Thanks a lot, Paige," I said, thinking about the fact that the longer I was at Shady Valley, the fewer pieces of mail I got. Of course, my friends sent cards to cheer me up, all ending with "thinking of you" and "keeping you in our prayers." But I used to be the queen of mail-order catalogs. I loved knowing the Loop was keeping up with the latest trends. It made me feel good, good about my store. I needed to order something besides a sweat suit to keep me on their lists.

Eventually, Paige said, "I better get them home. Do you need anything?"

"No, thanks, I'm set," I said, then remembered: "How'd Craig's show go?"

Paige smiled. "He was a hit. He even sold two of his big canvases. One to a local guy, and one to a New York collector who happened to be at the opening. He actually made some money. Can you believe it?" she gushed.

Paige was in love with a painter. Well, more than in love. Almost married to a painter named Craig, whose abstract art was about thirty years too late to be considered avant-garde. But still, he was gaining critical acclaim.

"That's great. Congratulations. Selfishly, I hope his career doesn't take off too fast, or you'll be leaving me for a studio in SoHo," I said, looking out the window and wondering what we'd do when Craig proposed and Paige left us.

Baby Hannah's drool puddled on my cheek and made me realize she was hovering over me, supported under her belly by Paige. I smiled. Paige said, "I'll see you again on Thursday. I'll ask Henry to bring them tonight too."

"Bye, Mommy. Sweet dreams," Hank said, blowing a kiss from the backseat of the double stroller. As Paige deposited her in the front seat, Hannah waved a balled-up fist in my general vicinity.

I'd take it. "Good-bye, babies," I said, and as usual, I had my cry.

When I was still at the hospital and not as weak as I was now, Hank was able to spend the night with me. That was before I was so weak. He'd pack his little suitcase with a lot of help from Paige, and he'd walk in wearing his feetie pajamas, carrying his teddy bear under his arm, and I just knew I would be OK. How could I not be OK with this perfect, tiny person to care for, to squeeze? With him cuddling me, life was a string of perfect moments.

3

Warning: If you generally consume three or more alcohol-containing drinks per day, consult your physician for when and how to take pain relievers.

MY FIRST PREGNANCY WAS SO EASY. LIFE CHANGED WITH OUR firstborn, of course. You don't realize how much time you waste in life until you have someone demand every spare moment. We went through a big change, Henry and I—individually and as a couple.

We both became less selfish. We had to. I had a business to run, and Henry was building his law career, but none of that mattered once Hank arrived. He came first. Before sleep. Before work. Before sex. My favorite memory of those crazy, firstborn newborn days was of Henry and me, exhausted, sneaking outside to talk—baby monitor in hand of course—so we would be sure not to wake Hank. We poured a couple glasses of wine and sat on our back porch step of our first house and both, finally, took a deep breath. It was August and a clear, steamy evening. The stars twinkled; a dog barked next door. Henry swore and swatted a mosquito. He was a magnet to mosquitos. Then we looked at each other, and we both started laughing. And we couldn't stop.

"You look horrible," Henry said, covering his mouth with one hand and fanning the air with the other, a human mosquito repellant.

"So do you," I said, tears streaming down my face, a release of all the worry and tension and newness a newborn brought to our life, our home.

"He's adorable. He has your lips," Henry said and leaned in for our first romantic kiss since we'd brought Hank home from the hospital. "And you're beautiful, as always."

"He has your eyes, I think," I said, kissing him back, in love with my husband and in love with our new family, even with the surging hormones and breasts full of milk.

"We're so lucky—*I'm* so lucky—to have you," Henry said. "Thank you for saying yes, and for picking me over Alex, over everybody else."

"It was never a choice. I loved you from the start, Henry," I said. Henry had a habit of bringing up Alex when he was in a reflective mood. I had a habit of changing the subject. There was no question in my mind. I had made the right choice. I loved my life with Henry, our new home complete with a perfect infant. Alex was my past; this was my future. As the baby monitor sprang to life with the cries of our little angel, we both smiled. Henry pulled me up from the step, and we hurried inside.

Of course I was thrilled when I discovered I was pregnant with Hannah. We'd overcome the stress of first-time parenting. The Loop was booming: it had become the local place for women to come and talk; to relax and shop; to drink wine, meet friends, gossip. And it was two blocks from home, in Grandville, the grandest ville around. Henry's business was booming too. We'd fall into bed at night next to each other, smile, kiss lightly on the lips, and race to see who could snore first. Full life. Fast life. Roses, all. And even though ten months of morning sickness followed, Hanna was meant to be a part of all that life.

As was my breast cancer. It would've developed sooner or later; it just got a big boost from my pregnancies. The doctors think my tumor began with Hank. After baby Hannah was born and after the fevers had come, the doctors suggested a mammogram. I stammered, "But I'm too young to have a mammogram. It doesn't run in my family. Where did this come from? Why me?"

That was later, after Hannah's birth. But first there was the reality of a growing baby boy in my home and the start of a second life inside me—happy times, except for the morning sickness. Looking back I wondered if it wasn't morning sickness at all but a more sinister signal that something was horribly wrong, a warning I was too busy to acknowledge.

My leap from advertising to entrepreneurship was less about faith and more about burnout. The pink-collar ghetto was getting to me. Really. Public relations was fine, as long you could figure out a way to be appreciated. The problem was the advertising folks got to spend all the money. Selling advertisements produced much more visible results than did trying to woo the editor of the metro section to do a business profile on your client, the world's largest refurbisher of industrial baking equipment, for example.

My boss, Milton, was a jerk. He was so consumed with becoming somebody important that he lost sight of everything else. On top of that, he was a sexist pig. One of his more memorable favorite activities was standing at the top of the office stairs on winter mornings, watching out the window, waiting to see who would slip and slide across the snow and ice to arrive late. Of course, none of us underlings could afford to park near the office, so it was a mad dash every morning.

"You're more than fifteen minutes late, Jennifer," he noted as I huffed in the door one morning. The night before we'd been stuck at the office working on a campaign until eight. That Saturday, we would all be working again.

I almost snapped but kept quiet. I'd just rented my first apartment, and Alex and I were on the rocks. I needed the job, and so I apologized to Milton. Obviously, I relished the times I could leave the office and head to a meeting. I dreamed about the day I'd be out on my own, with my own business, free of irritating bosses and their arbitrary rules. I didn't realize then that I was learning a lot from Milton and his ways, that I was growing a lot stronger. Strength I needed now.

After three years, I quit. Two months later, with a vote of confidence and a sizable loan from Daddy, I opened Clothes the Loop. Milton probably seethed about the amount of publicity I garnered for my store. I secretly hoped so. I selected a wonderful, old, brick building built in the 1920s in the heart of downtown Grandville, on the tree-lined Main Street. An outdoor café was to the left of my store, a hair salon to the right. Perfect.

People always asked me, "You're from a wealthy family, and Henry makes good money—why don't you just work at home? Do charity work like your mother does. Play tennis." The answer, for me, was that I just couldn't. While I had never known exactly what I wanted to become, I always knew I'd have a career. I had the burger king, my daddy, to thank for that. The firstborn, I basked in what little attention he gave his family while building his tiny burger chain into an empire. True, by the time I was in school, my pride in his success often served as a substitute for his actual presence, but I was undaunted in my admiration of him. I admired his tireless energy, his drive to succeed, and his power as a successful businessman, and I felt empowered by his example. I wanted to find something that excited me in the same way burgers got to Daddy. Most of all, I wanted him to be proud of me, I guess—to notice me.

I designed the interior of the Loop to showcase the designer clothes on the racks. The walls were painted a light beige, the floors were hardwood, and the dressing rooms in the back were large, with plush shag carpet for comfort. A small seating area with a couch and two chairs outside the dressing rooms encouraged my customers to stay and chat, enjoy a glass of wine. I loved my store, and I loved that its success verified my taste.

The best part about having my own business was making Hank a part of it. He came to work with me, slept in his portable crib, and charmed all of our customers. Jacob tolerated his presence, since he was a draw that led to higher sales. Often, at lunchtime, Henry would swing by, and the three of us would go to the country club. We were no longer the cold-shower couple of Maddie's column, but we were the happy couple, proud of our adorable son and of the life we were creating together.

I'd been careful not to gain too much weight with Hank, and I bounced back into my regular clothes quickly. "We need you to be the look of the Loop, Jenn, don't forget," Jacob had warned a bit snootily my first day back at the store with baby Hank in tow. He eyed my still-round midsection with distaste.

"Look, I'll be back in the saddle. I'm breast-feeding and—well, you don't want to know more, but don't worry about it. I'm back and better than ever," I added, convincing myself but not Jacob. His job was to be the cynic, and he excelled. We were a great balance—my overly optimistic, overly spunky demeanor versus his droll, snarky one.

Henry had worried, at first, about Hank being at the store, catching whooping cough or something else horrible from a sick customer. But after a few weeks, with regular lunches and frequent check-ins, he seemed relieved.

However, the lunches at the club had to stop once I became pregnant with Hannah. I couldn't stand the smell of food—except ribs and loaded baked potatoes. I was certain my daughter would never be a vegetarian.

This was the start of what Henry and I called my Martha Stewart phase. I was compelled to cook homemade dinners every night, resulting in an astronomical number of dirty bowls, pots, pans, and the like. Henry, being the designated dishwasher/cleaner-upper—a job he'd relished before Hank was born—was now the grumpy guy after dinner, wondering why takeout was fine for every other young family in Grandville.

"Homemade, organic—it's all important for Hank and now this other little one. Don't you want the best for your kids?" I'd say, provoking the silent treatment. As I walked up the stairs to give Hank his bath, I'd add, "I love you," from the top of the stairs, and Henry would always laugh. Sure, we were stressed, but life was full and happy.

When he finished cleaning up from the homemade meal, a tired Henry would join us in the nursery. The smell of baby powder and the sounds of soothing, mind-stimulating baby music would calm both Hank and Henry. We were a team, Henry and I. Dishes, babies, our home, our life. Partners. Friends. Laughing. Loving. Life wasn't perfect, but it was good.

Henry, Hank, and Hannah arrived right on time, and I was elated. I watched from my throne as Henry unpacked the kids' fast-food meals, setting them up with a picnic blanket on my floor. Hannah still used a bottle, so Henry carefully poured her apple juice into an empty one he'd brought. Hank grinned at me and said, "French fries, Mommy. Your favorite!"

"You're right, buddy. I hope Daddy brought me some," I said, smiling at Henry, hoping he'd notice my eyeliner and mascara and the bit of a smoky eye I'd created. "And I hope Grandpa doesn't catch us with another restaurant's fries!"

"Oh, Jennifer. You know there's not a Julie's on the way or I would have stopped. No one will ever have to know if we hurry and eat all the evidence, right, guys?" Henry said, his enthusiasm waning as he plopped into one of my brown chairs behind the kids. Poor guy—he was trying with the kids, but he seemed incapable of noticing whether I was smelly and ugly or clean with full makeup.

"Right, Daddy," Hank grinned, chomping on fries and playing with the toy car prize. Henry handed over his iPad to Hank, and the little guy took charge, picking out a show for his little sister and him to enjoy during their meal. Kids these days. So smart.

"You know, you look down today, honey. Anything wrong?" Henry said, walking across the room. "Hey, scoot over," he added, sliding into bed beside me. I tried to keep a space between us, to get his attention focused on me, on my face. But his body felt warm and solid. I was surprised how much I missed this, missed him. I felt myself move closer to him. I missed everything. I missed us. The kids. Even Elmo the stupid red puppet who was now singing to my kids. Did the fact he was blind to my attempts to look better, prettier, bother me? It must have.

Is anything wrong? Yes. No. Please notice my smoky eyes, my lip gloss. What matters? Where are we?

"I think it's just that now that the invitations are finished, I need to think of something else to do, to focus on, you know? I need to keep planning in order to keep being. Am I making sense?" I asked Henry.

"Sure. Let's plan a trip. A vacation. Just you and me. I've been thinking about it, even talked to a couple of your doctors. Chris is considering it. I mean, if you're game, I'd love for you to choose. We'll go wherever you'd like," Henry said, rubbing my head. I nuzzled in like a puppy dog. *I think that's a step above long-lost-uncle forehead kiss, but I'm not sure.* On the plus side, my husband wanted to go on vacation with me, so he must want to spend time with me. How wonderfully normal, how unexpectedly great. My heart swelled. I was a wife, with a husband who wanted to go on a vacation. Just the two of us. But—

"You'd have to do a lot of routine maintenance, you know, for me," I said, knowing he knew what I meant, since he'd taken care of me at home in between hospital stays, before I came to Shady Valley. This was the fear, the problem with me trying to imagine he could love me like he loved me before. As I shrunk under cancer's strain, nothing was the same. It was like the ad campaign for minivans: the smaller the person, the more space she occupies. The ad had a photo of all the stuff—car seat, playpen, stroller, walker, baby swing—the little person needed to travel. The smaller I got, the more equipment I needed.

"I know all about that. That's part of the pleasure of spending time with you," he said, joking. Seeing the look on my face, he quickly added, "Seriously, Jenn, give it some thought. We have time to plan a romantic and memorable trip together. OK? Oh, and you look really pretty tonight. I love how your hair is growing in curly."

"Do you think we could leave tomorrow?" I asked. *He noticed,* I thought. *My man loves me.*

"Why?"

"It will give me, us, something to look forward to, and I'm sick of being here, of course. I miss you, miss this," I said, snuggling into him. I looked up at him, hoping he'd lean down and kiss me, much like Ralph had. But he didn't.

"Well, I think you should tell me where you'd like to go, and I'll start planning it," Henry said, patting me on the head while rolling out of the bed. "Kids, it's time to get going, so let's practice cleaning up." Henry was a master at extraction. The youngest of four, Henry had successfully negotiated his own family dynamics by removing himself from his family's business, despite vehement protests from his dad. He went to law school and was just a year away from partnership at the law firm. It had been a much harder road for him to follow, but he had eventually earned his father's respect because of it.

He had the kids' picnic dinner cleaned up and both of them packed to leave before I could think of any reason to keep them in my room. Why did he have to hurry? Was I repulsive?

"Henry, Hank, Hannah—thank you for visiting tonight," I said.

Henry picked up Hannah, who gave me a kiss, and then Hank, who did the same. Henry patted me on the head and kissed my cheek. "Good night, sweetie, sleep tight," he said, pushing the stroller out the door before closing it softly in their wake.

I sat on the throne, pouting. Their visit, while wonderful, was too short. I looked around at the annoying green-striped walls and felt trapped. Trapped. Alone. Angry. I never was much of a demonstratively angry person—but I scanned the room for something to throw, to break. All I could find was my hairbrush, sitting on the bedside table. As I picked it up, I forced myself to breathe deeply, but still I wanted to throw it at something, and so I did—just as Ralph opened the door to my room with a quiet knock. The brush hit the opening door and ricocheted across the room, landing harmlessly on the floor.

"Ah, Jenn?" Ralph said, closing the door to a crack. "Are you still firing, or may I come in?"

I didn't answer, but he pushed open the door and made his way over to me.

"I heard Henry and the kids leaving and thought you might like some company. Or a good cry, or something," Ralph said, patting my hand, as I was indeed crying. "Look, you have hope. You'll make it out of here, you will. In the meantime, let's focus on healing instead of feeling sorry for ourselves. We can learn more about wine. And I'll focus on dreaming about kissing my wife—instead of my best friend," he added.

I chuckled despite myself.

And I'll stop dreaming about our kiss, and Alex, and my past and focus on my future, I thought, and willed myself to do just that.

4

Warning: Contents under pressure. Use extreme caution.

I watched as Julie carefully and slowly folded her purple umbrella, leaning it against the wall just inside my door. I was glad it rained. Maybe Ralph would get off his wine-and-sex kick. Maybe Julie would melt into the fake-wood floor of the valley of shade. Maybe she'd float away down the sea of green carpet. Maybe she'd just leave.

Then again, maybe she wouldn't.

My sister. She was a little shorter than me, maybe five feet four. Her hair was a rich chestnut like Daddy's, instead of my own ash-blond. Her eyes were a dark, deep blue, and her face was cherub round. The overall effect was that she was very innocent looking, even at thirty-one. She smelled like Juliana's Chanel, and she was wearing one of Juliana's cloud-gray outfits.

"Hi, Jennifer," she said, looking me over with overly sad eyes. "You are sooo thin." She did circle mouth. "Don't they feed you here? Do you want some fries or something? I could've stopped at Julie's on the way over," she said, tossing out her namesake restaurant while crossing the room to peer into my face. I saw puddles forming in the wake of her stylish ankle boots.

"No, I'm fine, thanks," I said tersely, pulling the covers up under my chin.

"Hey, you know Alex Thomas is single again," Julie said. She had perched cross-legged at the foot of my throne, all the better to see me in my dying splendor, and to gauge my startled reaction to her news. "He called the house, asked about you. Since I answered the phone, I felt I had to tell him the entire sad story about your cancer. He hadn't heard. He wants to visit you."

I stared. Could she be that cold? Was she testing me? Waiting for me to blush or swoon or something? *Alex is single again?* I was angered to feel my heart beating faster. I hoped she couldn't tell.

"He told me all about his wife. You know they were married for nine years, didn't have any kids? Get a load of that. I just looked at Mark, and I had a baby," Julie said, picking the polish off her newly manicured fingernails. Her left ring finger was missing its wedding ring. On her right ring finger she sported a ruby-and-diamond cocktail ring that had to be Juliana's, since it looked too prissy even for Julie. It also was far too expensive to be from her soon-to-be ex-husband, Mark.

Alex was single.

"Anyway, they separated a couple of months ago, so he's moving back up here, you know, from Dallas, 'cause he says the entire state of Texas reminds him of Cathy, and he needs a break." She paused. "Hello, are you going to talk at all?"

"Sure, what do you want to talk about?" I asked—too defensively.

"About Alex, of course. Your main squeeze. The love of your life, although Henry thinks he is." Julie smiled.

"Henry is the love of my life, Julie," I said.

"Right. Whatever. So should I tell Alex you'd like to see him, or not?"

"Of course I'll see him," I answered, careful to keep my voice breezy, my face expressionless. "He was going to get an invitation to my party anyway. But I guess he could come now. Sure, I could see him sooner," I said. Once I realized I was babbling, I stopped.

"Are you blushing?" Julie asked. "You are. He still turns you on, doesn't he?"

Bitch. "No, Julie, he doesn't. I cared about Alex for a long time, and I want to see him since he's in town—that's all," I answered righteously.

"He will be by this afternoon," she said smugly, standing up and turning her back to me. "So what's the deal with this party idea of yours? Mother is working herself to the bone on this project." She turned back around to face me. "Not that she isn't glad to be doing it for you, of course."

I ignored her. I was ticked. "Did you tell him to come by, that it was all right, before even asking me?" I demanded.

"Of course. Here's his number, if you need to reschedule. I told him four. That'll give you plenty of time. I mean, you've got six hours, if you start now. Or just call and cancel. So what's the deal with these parties you're hosting? I don't understand why you're doing it. What if you don't really die? Will people feel disappointed? Have you given up, Jenn?" Julie asked, looking sincere for once, her round face earnestly searching my thin oval one for the truth.

"No, I haven't given up, but I'm trying to be realistic. I guess, if I live, I mean, if I beat this thing, then I'll owe some people travel expenses or something. I hadn't really thought of a last-chance guarantee."

"Well, it just sounds like you're making light of your chances and all," Julie said.

"Julie, if it weren't for Shady Valley, I probably wouldn't even be here now. I've been on borrowed time for a while now, so I'm definitely not making light of anything." Changing the subject, I asked, "How are my girls?" I loved my sister's kids purely. Children could do no wrong in my eyes, even if they belonged to some of the most self-centered adults I knew. Kids were innately good; it was adults who spoiled them and made them bad. Lillie and Riley were still too young to be anything but innocent, although my sister and my mother would probably eventually corrupt them. By age ten, they'd be intolerable, I felt sure.

"They're adorable. Riley told me to tell you thanks for the Barbie. She wanted to come, but I didn't know how you'd look—you know, if you'd scare her or whatever. I think she should come," Julie said, appraising my appearance. "You know, except for the dark circles under your eyes, you really look good. A little thin, but that's always in. With the right makeup and some soft lights, Alex will kick himself for letting you get away."

Alex again.

Prom our senior year was the first time we came close. It wasn't a matter of if we'd have sex—it was a matter of when. We'd been together more than a year, and Alex had been patient. I had wanted to wait until college—for no other reason than the fact high school was full of rumors, and I just didn't want to be included. I knew I could trust Alex, but I wasn't sure I could trust myself. I'd tell a friend if we "did it." I knew I would.

Alex picked me up that warm spring night. Eventually our group would meet for preprom dinner at a new restaurant downtown, one where the servers would card us as soon as we walked in sporting our boutonnieres and corsages. So we headed first to a dive motel. Alex had reserved the room, and he and his friends had stocked it with booze. I wore a dark-purple midcalf dress and high heels, my hair painstakingly curled and loose. As I sipped my champagne and posed for photos with our friends, Alex smiled and gave me a wink. Always, he watched me. I found it comforting. He loved me so much.

We stayed at the prom long enough to dance one dance and smile at Mr. Cooper, the principal. We snuck out the back, the way generations of Grandville seniors had, and headed back to the motel room.

"Where is everybody else?" I asked, my head still light from the champagne.

"They are going elsewhere, Jenn. This is our room tonight," he answered, taking my hand and pulling me onto one of the two queen beds.

"But," I said, before I realized there was nothing I could say. My parents knew I was out for the evening, supposedly spending the night at Betsy's. "Alex, you know I want to wait."

"Shhhh," he said, slowly kissing me on my neck as he expertly removed my dress. "You are gorgeous," he said, quickly unfastening my bra and releasing my breasts. I felt dizzy, and wonderful, and in love—and I wanted him, wanted this more than anything else. My rules were arbitrary, and everyone was doing it.

"Alex, yes," I said.

He really wasn't trying to force me. He stopped, looked into my eyes, and asked, "Are you sure?"

I had nodded yes.

I realized Julie was still talking. "You won't believe how big Riley is now." Her voice was always softer when she talked about her girls. "I can't believe she's already four. She acts fourteen, of course. And with Mark's wild, curly, black hair—she's like the Tasmanian devil. I can't control it, so I don't even try anymore. Oh, you have to see the precious matching outfits I got them at the Bal Harbour Oilily last time I was in Miami. Brown-and-white cow-spot leggings, brown-and-white checked tops, white patent leather purses, the works. They looked like little endangered species flying home on the plane," Julie said, laughing at the memory. "I mean, remember those days, Jenn, when Mother made us dress alike?"

I did remember those days. Mother and Julie trying to outshine each other. Julie and I wore matching outfits that somehow always made her look sweet while I looked awkward.

"That sounds like fun, Julie," I said, growing tired from the effort that talking to her always required. Deep down I knew I loved her, but after a lifetime of feeling competed with, I found her wearing. I loved her, but I didn't trust her.

Sensing my mood, Julie grabbed her Louis Vuitton purse to leave.

"Anyway, I need to get going. When you'd like me to visit again, just call the house. I'll be in Grandville for a while, just sorting things out. Mind you, I'm taking my time. I didn't realize how great we had it growing up until I tried to make a home of my own. It's tough. And expensive and not as nice as Mommy and Daddy's place."

"That's because we grew up in a mansion, Julie, with other people taking care of everything for us. Welcome to the real world. Oh, and thanks for talking to Alex. It'll be good to see him," I said, the understatement of the day. *It was going to be awesome seeing him*, I thought.

"Yes, I've had fun getting caught up with him too. He's still so cute," Julie said and smiled. "You really shouldn't have let him get away, Jenn. Don't you regret it at all?"

"I'm so lucky with my life now, even with cancer. I hope you'll find happiness and get back on your feet soon. Good luck with everything, Julie," I added seriously. She would be fine. She always was, once the drama subsided.

"Thanks, Jennifer. Get well," she said, her chunky heels tapping across my floor. Gracefully, she bent down and picked up her still-wet purple umbrella, gave a quick wave, and was gone.

I forgot to ask Julie what Mother thought about the invitations. *Drat*. Now I had to call her.

"You know, darling, I still find the entire notion a bit macabre, but if you insist, we'll still do it for you," Juliana said to me over the telephone. "I showed it to your father last night and he just, well, he looked so sad. So—"

"I know he feels bad because I'm dying," I said. "Did you tell him to visit already?"

"Not dying, dear. You're sick—very sick. But we're not finished fighting yet. Did Julie bring the painting in?" Mother asked.

"What?" I asked. She was changing topics so fast I was having trouble keeping up.

"Oh, I found a gorgeous landscape, perfect for that barren wall behind the ugly brown chairs. She was supposed to bring it in to you."

"She didn't, but I'm sure she's arranging for someone else to bring it in for her, if it was loaded into her car," I answered, sounding sarcastic and mean. I couldn't help it. Julie was lazy.

"It was; she drove my car," Mother said, sounding as if she were growing tired of this conversation too.

"Thanks, Mother, for everything. I'll talk to you tomorrow," I said, hanging up.

"Jennifer? You missed breakfast, so I really think you should try some lunch," the college candy striper said, whispering next to my bed. I must've fallen asleep.

"What time is it?" I asked, suddenly panicked. Alex was coming.

"It's about a quarter to three," Stripes answered.

"Oh no. Yes, thanks, leave the lunch. I need to get ready, fast. Can you help?" I hated to ask for a hand, but this was an emergency. I had a little over an hour of primp time to prepare for the man who used to be the love of my life. Julie was right about that.

"Yes, that one," I said to Stripes as she held up one of my favorite sweat suits. She brought it to me as I felt a sharp stab of guilt from my conscience. Yellow. Soft. Flattering. Henry loved me in yellow.

By the time I was dressed and feeling as pretty as I could get, it was 4:10. No Alex. Maybe it was all a Julie joke. *No disappointment,*

Jennifer, I said to myself. *Heck, I haven't seen the guy in eight years, almost as long as we dated. It's so over. He's probably fat or bald or mean or ugly or—*

"Hey, Jennifer," Alex said, knocking on the door of my room. "Up for a visitor?"

"Sure," I answered My heart was racing, and my palms were sweating. He hadn't changed. Not at all. He wasn't fat or bald or wrinkled or mean looking. No, he looked just like Alex. Mysterious. Strong. Refined. He walked over to the throne, which felt very much like a hospital bed right then, and kissed me lightly on the top of the head.

"I've missed you, Jennifer," he said. "It's been too long."

Say something lighthearted, my brain was screaming, but my mouth wouldn't do it. My heart was Thumper the rabbit. I sat mute. An eternity passed before I managed to chirp, "I've missed you too. Life goes so fast."

"For being as sick as everybody says you are, you sure do look beautiful," Alex said.

"I am pretty sick, Alex," I said, agreeing for once with everybody, "but I'm so glad you can visit. Have a seat. Can you stay a while?"

"Absolutely," he said, walking over to the brown chair on the left—everybody's favorite. I thought he'd sit, but he didn't. Instead, he picked up the ugly thing and carried it over next to the bed. I was still floating above him but not by too much. I scrunched down so we'd be more eye to eye. I was almost lying flat.

Once he was close to me, and I caught a whiff of his smell, suddenly my body was screaming to be touched, to be kissed passionately and not chastely on the forehead. The air was electric with our unspoken feelings, and I knew he felt that too. Our eyes were locked.

"Seriously, you are so cute," he said, reaching over and rubbing my head. *Really? You too,* I thought. It wasn't exactly the passion-swept embrace of my dreams, but I was a married woman, after all. *What am I thinking?*

"So, Gorgeous, I heard all about your successful store and your two kids. Julie filled me in. I also know the cancer is pretty aggressive. But you're gonna beat it, Jenn. I know you are. You have too many people pulling for you, and besides, you look too good." I wanted to believe every word he said. I used to. I had trusted Alex to be the man I made love to for the first time. I trusted him to be my prom date, my best friend, my driving teacher, and even my drug pusher the first time I smoked pot. I had believed we'd always be together then.

Sadly, so had Alex.

"I hope you're right, but I'm afraid it's pretty bad," I said. "I've turned on myself, so to speak. It's some sort of deep, dark mutiny in my cells. And the doctors won't cut it out—it's too advanced for that. But I'm not giving up, Alex, not yet."

Alex reached over and took my hand. "Of course you're not giving up," he said. "You will beat this. We will beat this. I'm here, whatever you need."

His brown eyes filled with tears, and soon mine did too. I pulled my hand away from his to wipe my eyes. I couldn't lean on him, on the past. I couldn't go back to this, to what I was, what we were.

"Tell me about your life," I said in a blatant attempt to change the subject.

Alex shook his head and wiped his eyes with one quick swipe of his right hand. His eyes didn't hold the pity I usually saw reflected in visitors. They held something far deeper.

"Hey, it's OK, I'm OK. Talk to me," I said gently.

Alex's eyes came back into focus, and he gave me a wide smile. I tried another question to break the silence. "Fill me in. Why are you back in town?" I asked innocently, as if I didn't know about his separation.

"Things didn't work out with Cathy, Jennifer. You know she was the first girl I dated after we broke up. I'm not sure I ever really loved her. Not like I loved you."

He looked at me with his dark eyes, and I felt my heart lurch. Handsome and lovely Alex. Did he still want me, even now?

"You know, Jennifer, we could've decided that night to do it. To spend the rest of our lives together, instead of breaking up forever, I mean," Alex said, looking down and back up, his eyes full of meaning.

"At least you won't be the one getting short changed by my premature demise," I said nervously, trying to sound chipper even as my heart raced. Sure, it was great to realize my first love still loved me. But, it didn't mean anything, not now, not anymore. It couldn't. It didn't.

"That's not funny. The worst part is the time we wasted when we should have been together. It would've been fantastic, just like we always dreamed of."

"Jennifer?" a familiar voice interrupted.

Henry was standing in the doorway.

Alex jerked upright. Startled, I thought, *Perfect. Henry sounds mad; did he hear our conversation?*

"Henry, hi, I'd like you to meet Alex Thomas, an old friend of mine," I stammered, trying to sit higher up in my throne. Of course, everyone who everyone was. My head was spinning again, but this time I couldn't blame the cancer.

"I thought you lived in Texas now, Alex," Henry said, overanimatedly shaking Alex's hand. I hoped Henry didn't squeeze so hard he would crush Alex's hand.

"Actually, I did. Until just recently. I've moved back to town for a spell," Alex said.

For a spell? I wondered. *And why is Henry here?*

"Still married?" Henry asked.

"Nope. Unfortunately, Cathy became hopelessly enthralled with an oil-baron type. She couldn't resist all that flashy money." Alex said, shaking his head. His own family had plenty of "flashy money," and I suspected there was much more to the story than Alex wanted to share. "We never took the time to have any kids, so at least there's that to be grateful for."

Henry settled on the end of the bed. "We're so lucky. We have two great kids, a lot of family around for moral support, and Jennifer is getting better by the day. Right, honey?" Henry asked as he leaned forward and gave me an awkwardly long, sloppy kiss on the lips.

"Absolutely," I said, fighting the urge to wipe my mouth with the back of my hand. *Really? Our first kiss in forever was only to mark his territory?* This was like a bad dream. My first love. My husband. Squaring off over my sick bed. A movie of the week. Perhaps they could have a duel or host a cockfight later, just to finish things off.

"Is it still raining?" I asked lamely, to no one in particular. The warm, yellow night was clearly visible through the window in my room, matching the color of my sweat suit.

"No, honey, it stopped a couple of hours ago," Henry answered, rubbing my feet through the sheet.

The silence grew louder as I searched in vain for some neutral topic to discuss. "If it's all right with you guys, I'd like to stop by and visit again soon," Alex said, standing to leave. "Unless you'd rather—"

"Yes, please do, Alex," I said, ignoring that Alex was obviously speaking to Henry. I kept my eyes averted from Henry's face while he also answered.

"She'd enjoy the company, Alex. I can only be here so often, with the kids and my practice. Another visitor would be great," Henry said, only the slightest hesitation in his voice.

"Great, then, good night. I'll see you soon," Alex said as he shook Henry's outstretched hand. He nodded in my direction and then hustled out of the room.

"That must've been a surprise," Henry said. "Unless you knew ahead of time?"

"It seems he called the house and got the scoop from Julie about my cancer. He felt sorry for me, I guess, and showed up," I answered. "Anyway, how was your day?"

"Any regrets, Jennifer?" Henry asked in a serious tone.

"What do you mean?" I asked, forcing myself to meet his gaze, knowing exactly what he was asking. Did I have regrets? Did I make the right choice? Of course I did. Of course. But it was nice to be told I was attractive by a man, to be looked at in that way again.

"I mean about us. Do you regret marrying me?" he said, his blue eyes locking with mine, the foot massage now suspended.

"Of course not. I still can't believe how lucky I am to be married to you," I said, smiling. And it was true.

From the moment I first saw Henry, I was infatuated, and Maddie had watched it all unfold. She and I were at a government reception. She was gathering scoop for her gossip column, and I was still working at an advertising agency in town. We'd become friends despite the fact I was constantly pitching her stories about my clients.

She called and invited me to go to an after-work event in honor of a park being created along the riverfront. As we emerged upstairs into a crush of thirsty VIPs, I spotted him. Henry.

It was love at first sight. For me, anyway. He was tall, blond, square chinned, spunky. Henry made my palms sweat. It didn't hurt that Alex and I were on one of our downswings.

"Maddie, I've got to meet that guy," I said, grabbing her arm and nodding across the ice sculpture in Henry's direction.

"That guy is Henry Benson Jr., heir to the Grandville Company fortune, and a complete wild man, from what I hear," Maddie said, her dark-brown eyes conspiratorially scanning the crowd. "He's unattached, very eligible, and an attorney, to boot. We should go talk to him," she added, firing up a Marlboro Light.

I didn't even think about her breaking the law. "What if he hates smoking?" I asked her, panicked he'd be turned off of me by association.

"Then we'll know he's no fun and a prude," she answered, blowing a column of smoke into the air. In her trademark all-black suit, she looked like the smoke stack of a steam engine—the little engine that could. I waited for someone from the hotel to ask her to extinguish it. No such luck—just a few nasty stares from fellow party attendees as we cut through the crowd.

We approached Henry's social cluster by rounding the large buffet table. It was amazing how many people knew Maddie, and they looked at me to see if I was a trailing photographer from the newspaper, hoping to have their photos on the society party page. My boss, Milton Lester, lived to see his mug there. That was my primary job at the ad agency: Milton Lester's personal publicity.

And suddenly, we were talking to Henry. Well, Maddie was talking. I was nodding. Henry was grinning. And then Maddie was gone, and I was staring into his eyes, and I could've charged a power plant with the electricity coursing through my system. And we were leaving the reception, and we were riding down the escalator, and we were outside.

Henry and me.

"Would you like to go to dinner sometime?" he asked.

"I'd love to," I answered. I was flushed. Bright, neon red, like a tanning-bed burn.

"How about Thursday night? Lindey's? Seven thirty?" he was saying.

I swooned, right there on the corner of Broad and High. I couldn't remember where I'd left my car.

Thursday had seemed forever away. Time moved slowly back then. At twenty-six, I still thought it was endless. Milton had watched me at the party and teased me all week about my flirting.

I didn't tell him about dinner. I asked Maddie to put him in her column that week to get him off my back. She did, and Milton backed off.

I don't know what we ate on our date, and Henry could never remember either. After, he walked me to my car and waited until I sat down in the driver's seat and closed the door. I rolled down the window, and he bent his head down, and I turned my cheek. I was dating Alex, officially, but Henry was exciting. I couldn't kiss his lips, not yet.

He smiled down at me then in the light from the street lamp.

"Sorry, I just—" I stammered.

"Don't worry about it, Jennifer. I had a great time tonight. Good night." He turned and walked away.

Now my knight in shining armor was asleep next to me on the throne. Snoring. A single-parent, business-owning knight, who still managed a tinge of jealousy when his dying wife's former lover was at her bedside.

How could I have let myself get carried away by the sight of Alex, even for a second? Our past together was marred by deceit and painful breakups. Alex and I could never stay truly happy together, never truly right, once we went off to college. We were simply high school sweethearts who went on hurting each other long past the time other couples had gone their separate ways.

Truth be told, it was mostly my fault. I just wasn't ready to settle down, not when there were four years of college to be lived. One night, freshman year, I had my roommate talk to Alex. Mary tried to explain to him why it would make sense for us to date other people. Why it was important.

"There are so many date parties here," Mary explained, with the simple truth and a sweet Southern drawl.

Alex, on speaker phone, sighed and said, "There are date parties here too, Mary. Jenn, I know I'm on speaker. I can fly down there whenever you need me to be your date. And you know I want you

It was midmorning when Ralph hobbled in, looking better than thought he would. I'd spent my morning watching repetitive news gments, playing with my breakfast, and writing in my journal. ong ago I'd stopped searching the Internet, looking for information out my disease. It was too disheartening. Instead, I wrote when I d extra energy. I smiled and closed the journal when I saw him.

He said, "It's crushing time in the wine country. At least for rtain grapes." He sat on one of the chairs. "I've been reading a lot the subject, and it seems something called crushing technology s replaced stomping grapes with one's bare feet, just so you know."

I told him, "Stomping sounds more fun."

He rolled his eyes in his inimitable fashion. I loved it when he d life in those eyes, and that this morning's public fight with arbara hadn't seemed to crush his spirit. But still, crushing sounded inful. Stomping sounded spirited. Crushing reminded me of the adaches. Of the garish, fluorescent-lit hallways of the hospital here my cancer was diagnosed. Of the pulsing, beeping, scurrying, efficient, chaotic atmosphere of the emergency room. Of being side an MRI for an hour, in a metal canister, with a jackhammer work all around you. That was crushing. Grapes, though, whether ardonnay, merlot, pinot, or whatever, deserved to be stomped, if u asked me. Nature's candy.

"Did you know when you squeeze a grape, whether its skin is d, purple, or green, the juice is clear?" Ralph asked.

"Nope, didn't know that, great Bacchus," I answered. "Seriously, alph, what's with this new hobby of yours?"

"Pure, pointless pleasure," he answered.

"Sounds good, actually—please continue," I said.

He smiled. I thought, *Maybe I should arrange a wine tasting at hady Valley. We could decorate the lobby like a winery, hang some grapes, t pitchers of sparkling water and dry crackers, loads of wine, obviously, d invite an expert to explain all those high-brow things about wine*

here whenever you can be for my fraternity parties. Come on, Jenn, keep Mary out of this. I could be down there tonight. I'm not doing anything this weekend."

I imagined Alex sitting outside his dorm room, frustrated and alone. Meanwhile, I couldn't wait to get off the telephone and go out. What was wrong with me? Was it because he was so committed he scared me? I didn't know, but I knew I couldn't deal with this conversation.

"Alex, look, I love you, and I love us. But during the school year, we agreed to see other people. Please enjoy college and let me enjoy it too," I said firmly. Mary gave me a thumbs-up.

"You go enjoy, Jenn. I'll be here," he said and hung up.

Alex. Maybe if he hadn't been so nice, I wouldn't have taken him for granted. But if we had been meant to be, wouldn't we have been? By sophomore year, I'd started lying to Alex about who I was dating, because I was dating. And all of my roommates became part of the cover-up. It was for his own good, I thought. And they all agreed.

Still, at Shady Valley, I couldn't pretend I hadn't felt a charge between us. I glanced across the room and saw the landscape from my mother leaning against the wall. New things were appearing everywhere. As I drifted off to sleep, I smiled, knowing I would undoubtedly see him again.

5

Warning: Do not overfill or mound.

IT WAS 9:00 A.M., ACCORDING TO MY LARGE SPEAKERPHONE/CLOCK, when I awoke to Barbara's angry words floating down the hall, even though I tried to block them out. My door was open because it was a hot fall day.

"We can't, Ralph. You can't go anywhere…The doctors, that's who," she yelled.

I imagined Ralph imploring her to come inside his room, to talk quietly. I knew he valued the scant privacy he still had, the slim honor that came from keeping your family life private when everything about your body wasn't. My heart ached for him, for them. My ears had become huge, attuned to every sound coming from the hallway. They didn't need to work that hard, though.

"Are you crazy? Do you want to kill yourself? God, a trip! A trip!" Barbara said, her voice oscillating in loudness as if she were turning her head back in forth. Perhaps she was shaking it in disgust? There was silence, and I hoped she had gone inside his room. She hadn't.

"Oh yes, and this is a walk in the park for me and the kids. We are loving every minute, every bill, every phone call, every fucking

pitiful stare from people we thought were our friends! L And I didn't tell you about the house because there isr you can do about it. It's gone, Ralph. Everything is gor

Hadley shut my door on her way past my room. I I closing in her wake and imagined her barreling towa forcing her into Ralph's room, or out the front door. H be mean—she could be tough on us patients—but she tolerate this, this unthinkably raw pain coursing dow green hallway of Shady Valley.

Soon, everything was quiet. I turned on the news restless. I had to go check on Ralph. I opened my door, and looked for Hadley, who was nowhere to be seen. Slo my way down the carpeted hallway and paused just outs partially opened door. As I was about to enter, I notic standing just inside the door, quietly sobbing.

"Barbie, I know this is tough on you, I know," Ra couldn't see him, but imagined him sitting on the edge From the strain in his voice, I could tell he was crying

"No, Ralph, you don't know, you could never know. to hold it together, but I can't. I can't take it anymore," B Her right hand held the doorknob, and her long finge painted a bright red.

"I know you need space, time. Take as much as you promise you'll be back, with the kids. I need you," Ral My heart sank as tears formed in my eyes. I felt like and rescuing him. I felt like turning and running back to

"Good-bye, Ralph," Barbara announced as she sudc through the door and raced past me down the hall.

The sound of Ralph's sobs followed me as I made m to my room.

while the residents simply got wasted. Maybe I'd put Juliana in charge of that event—after my party, of course. That way, Ralph and Barbara could get away to the wine country without going anywhere.

"You know what I find fascinating? Even with all the technology, all the huge wineries, the grapes are still picked, bunch by bunch, by hand," Ralph said, staring at his large, thin hands. *Those fingers should play the piano,* I thought. *Those fingers should be playing with his wife's hair, holding her hand.*

"Even with technology, there's only so much control we have over nature. We're proof of that, aren't we?" I said, looking down at my own hands. My fingers should be bathing my children, making a mess in the kitchen in a Martha Stewart way. But we had been, both of us, randomly selected to have our cells turn against us. Something in our genetic makeup, controlled by nature, chose the time and place to deliver us cancer.

"Some of the vineyards are beginning pesticide-free growing experiments. That's going to really benefit our kids' generation," Ralph said, shifting his stare to me. "Without all that shit—chemicals, preservatives, and all that—we might never have gotten sick, Jennifer. Just one of those nasty substances could've done it, triggered a cell revolt."

"We'll never know."

"No, we won't. Ergo, we drink wine," Ralph said with a smile.

"Sounds great. I'll have Henry bring a bottle tonight. You and Barbara can join us. What flavor?" I asked, and he flinched.

"We had a fight this morning, Jenn. I'm not sure we'll be talking anytime soon," he said, turning away from me. "And wine is not a flavor, as you know—it's an experience."

"OK, maybe you could call her, explain you want to get drunk on wine, and the only person you'd like to do that with is her, if she can spare the evening. A date. Sort of. Call her, Ralph. You miss her," I urged. "You just need to give each other a break."

"I do miss her, but doesn't she have the right to take a break from all of this?" he asked, looking up at me then with dark-brown, tear-rimmed eyes. "She came here this morning, and we had a terrible fight. Worst one ever."

"I'm sorry," I said, wondering if I should let him know that we all knew, heard the fight, and that I had tried to come to his rescue, standing just outside his door. "Maybe it's not about flying to the wine country. Maybe you just need a night away from here. Go anywhere. A bed-and-breakfast. Just a change of scenery." I didn't think there were any more experimental treatments coming his way. If not, why not?

"Maybe they'd let me out, you know, but I don't know how Barbara would handle it, my being a virtual invalid and all," Ralph sighed.

"That's for her to decide. You need to decide if you can handle it out there, in the real world, in a wheelchair. Handle the looks, the silent pity, the stares. If you can, then cheers," I said.

"I don't much care about the stares from strangers anymore, Jennifer," Ralph said, standing slowly, holding on to the arm of the brown chair. "It's the stares from Barbara that hurt the most now."

"You know what I just read, Ralph?" I asked, trying to change the subject. "In the 1930s, only one in five cancer patients was alive five years after diagnosis. In the forties it was one in four; in the sixties, only one in three; and in 2010 it was one out of two-and-a-half patients who got cancer was alive five years after diagnosis. And I was diagnosed only last year, and you too. So I figure, you and me, we'll make it; we'll be around. We can last, if we don't give up."

"What's your point?" he asked, beginning to shuffle slowly to my door with his walker.

"Follow your heart, Ralph, before it's too late," I said, and he nodded in agreement as he turned down the green hall.

It wasn't the time for indecision and hopelessness, not for us. If he wanted beluga caviar, fresh from the Caspian Sea, he should eat it, today. While climbing Mt. Everest might be out of our reach, other dreams weren't. Not yet. If he wanted to stomp grapes, or roll over them in his wheelchair, he should. A trip could renew his spirits.

Also, according to a story I read in the paper about a study of middle-aged men, those who felt hopeless or thought of themselves as failures were at greater risk of developing atherosclerosis, a narrowing of the arteries leading to heart attack or stroke. The article said people who showed high levels of despair had a 20 percent increase in artery clogging in four years, the same as resulted from smoking a pack a day. Giving up had strong negative consequences.

As everybody at Shady Valley knew, hopelessness spelled death. I had seen it. You gave up, either because of the pain or because a loved one turned her back on you, and you died. Poof. I refused to let that happen to Ralph. Or me. I'd be sure Jacob brought some wine when he came to see me.

Thursday afternoon was his visit time. I called the store's voice mail and left word for him to bring half a case of wine, any kind, that afternoon. I knew the wine and Jacob would cheer Ralph. Ralph liked Jacob. Jacob made other people feel good. I considered him family. We fought. We teased. We supported. I loved his visits as much as I loved working with him at our store. His snarky sense of humor, along with his true gift of fashion sense, made us a great team. It was our store. When I founded Clothes the Loop, I saw it as a reflection of me. And it still was, but it had become so much more. It was Jacob DuPry's too, and he deserved a lot of credit for the growing success over the last year. Sometimes I had to fight back a jealous pang. I knew I'd be welcomed back as soon as I recovered. Today I didn't allow the word "if" to creep in, although it hovered in the corner just out of reach, taunting me always.

We had grown a business from nothing into the most successful clothing boutique in the city. Jacob helped me have it all. Not that juggling career and family was ever easy, but Jacob made it possible.

When I first hired him to manage the Loop, I thought of him as an employee. That lasted about a month. It all changed one day with Gymboree. When Hank was six months old, I had rushed to meet him and Paige, his newly hired nanny, at his first Gymboree class. I raced in the door, late as I was for virtually everything in those days, ducked into the bathroom, and changed into sweats. I folded my gray designer pants carefully, since I needed to go back to the store right after class. Joining Paige and Hank in the circle, I sat down just as the teacher asked how many of the mommies in the class worked outside the home. I was the only one who raised my hand. All of the other women stared at me. Next, the teacher asked who *got* to stay home full time. The rest then raised their hands.

"Oh how wonderful," the teacher said. "When I have kids, I'm staying home full time. I could never leave my precious baby for somebody else to raise. Now, let's start with 'Row, Row, Row Your Boat.' Put your little one on the floor in front of you—that's it—rock forward and back. That's right…"

By the time I got back to the Loop, I was more mad than sad. Jacob helped plot my revenge on Gymbo the Clown for the rest of the day, and pretty soon, he had me laughing in spite of myself.

"I just can't do this, this half-in and half-out thing. You should have seen me with the parachute at the end of class. I swear, every one of those other mommies was out to mess up my hair," I whined.

"Just forget about that place. Now, really, Jennifer. Wouldn't Hank get more out of some quiet time alone with you than with some know-it-all clown exploiting nursery rhymes? He's a *baby*, for crying out loud!"

I got immense satisfaction from my Gymboree refund, and I kept my Tuesday morning dates with Hank, minus the pompous clown. I thanked Jacob for that.

I smiled as Jacob burst into my room. It was our standing Thursday afternoon date, and he was as happy as I'd seen him in months. "You're not going to believe the sales yesterday!" Another plus: he was hoisting a case of wine. "A record-setting day yesterday, and today, as a matter of fact. An almost perfect day, except for that ridiculous Katherine Jenkins. She's an immature spoiled brat. I can't take her. She had me running back and forth like a servant. I wish you could still handle her for me. Oh well, once you're back you will, right? Please," he begged.

I remembered when customers used to frazzle me. How I longed for those days.

"She doesn't bother me, particularly since she spends at least three thousand dollars every time she drops in. It's worth an hour of suffering. Who else came in?" I asked as Jacob unfolded the butterfly chair, yellow, that he kept in the corner of my room, behind the high chairs. He hated fake brown leather. Said he wouldn't be caught dead sitting on those gnarly beasts.

"Let me see if you can guess," Jacob said, settling in to do another one of his awful impressions. "Jennifer, darling, are you all right? You look drawn, you're melting away like butter," began Jacob in his imitation. According to Jacob, all suburban women over thirty sounded like Barbara Walters with a cold. I told him that—but it didn't deter him one bit. "Oh, well, back to me. I must find something suitable for the museum ball, but Jacob just couldn't seem to help. I know you will, right? Mother says you have the best eye. Has Rhonda been in yet? When she does, she snatches up all my sizes. I was thinking something pastel and flowing, yet clingy, you know. I don't work out five days a week to cover up this body." Jacob paused in his impersonation to uncork the bottle of chardonnay he'd extracted from the box. What the heck, it had to be past four.

OK, I'd play along. "Susan. Relax. I have just the dress for you," I said in my best placating tone. "Jacob, be a darling and bring our favorite customer a glass of our finest wine. Katherine, you go on back into the dressing room, and I'll be right there. I could bring you a paper bag, and you'd look fabulous. The addition to your house looks spectacular, by the way. You'll be the talk of Grandville, the biggest home on Berkshire Road."

"Perfect! Bravo! You still know how to suck up when you have to," Jacob said, popping the cork.

"Thanks for bringing the wine. Did you bring any stemware?"

"Is my butterfly chair adorable?" Jacob said as an answer and produced two crystal wine glasses from the wine box. "God, that's an awful landscape," he added, looking over the newest work of art now gracing my wall, compliments of Nurse Hadley and her hammer and nail.

"From Mother. I think it kind of looks like Northern California, if you squint your eyes and tilt your head."

"It looks even more like that if you close your eyes. Cheers," he said, handing me my glass. "Your message said you needed wine. For you? Or is there another poor person in need of alcohol?"

"Ralph could really use a glass. And thanks, Jacob."

"No problem. I'll go over, see if he's up to joining us. I'll be right back," Jacob said, and he was out the door. I took the time to sip my wine slowly and was surprised at how easily it went down. I loved the feeling of real crystal in my hand, and I swirled the wine, playing with the light caramel liquid that left its legs running down the inside of the crystal bowl. It was smooth and tasted so good. If Jacob didn't return soon, I'd have to shuffle over for more.

To my delight, and surprise, just then Daddy showed up in my doorway. "How's my number one daughter doing today?" *Daddy, at last.* He was wearing his favorite golf getup and a rather fake smile. His silver hair glistened in the fluorescent hallway light.

"Daddy," I said, thinking I sounded more ten than thirty-four. "I'm so glad you're here." And I was. The fact that the person I felt closest to in my entire family happened to be an emotionally distant workaholic didn't bother me at times like these. Only later. Right now, as always when he showed up in person, Daddy was firmly perched on his pedestal.

"Jennifer, my love," he said, pausing for a moment at the sight of the yellow butterfly chair and then graciously ignoring it and perching on the edge of the throne. "We can beat this thing. I was talking to my friend—you remember Dr. Jones at the Anderson? He suggested another trip to Houston."

"Oh, Daddy, you know there's nothing else they can do at MD Anderson that they're not doing here. Dr. Chris is in touch with those guys all the time. I'm on the latest trial. It's working."

"Well, it better be, darling, it better be. I just want the best for you, and I can make it happen. I don't like you being here, not at all," he said, shaking his head, unaccustomed to being out of control, without power over a situation.

A few months ago, Daddy had broken down in my hospital room, because he couldn't fix everything for me. Couldn't make everything OK. Even he couldn't make the cancer go away. I had cried too, but not for myself.

"Why can't they get this damn thing under control?" he had said to Nurse Hadley, who'd interrupted our visit by walking in to check my vitals.

She looked startled that he'd addressed her; they'd never talked before, as far as I knew. "Sir, she is getting the best care available," Hadley answered in her professional voice, quickly rolling up the blood pressure cuff and heading toward the door.

Daddy had gone into my bathroom, giving us both time to compose ourselves. Once he came back, he said, "Why, I believe I scared her off. Did you see how fast she skedaddled out of here?" He'd dried his tears and came to stand next to the throne, putting his hand on my shoulder. "I just want answers. I know you do too, honey. It's just the darnedest thing." His blue eyes filled again, and he turned away.

"Daddy, it's going to be OK," I had told him, wanting to believe it, for both of us. "This new treatment really seems to be working. I'm getting out of here soon. I just know it. Want to watch TV?" I pushed the remote, and we watched a comedy about nothing. It seemed the perfect anecdote to that visit, when we'd run out of things to say.

Now, I reminded him again that I knew he was doing the best he could. "I know, and thank you. I'm getting better—I can feel it. So where have you been, anyway? I've missed you. How's the burger business?" I asked, hopefully changing the subject.

"Great, really. Our sales weren't affected much by that E. coli scare," he answered in his businessman voice, ignoring the first question. "Our reputation stands for something at Julie's. Meanwhile, I still need to find a number two, even though I always figured it would be you," he said, his blue eyes betraying the sadness his smile tried to hide.

His face seemed older, more wrinkled than just a week before. And when he reached for my hand, I noticed the age spots on his. The farmer's tan from golf was typical, but all in all, my invincible daddy was beginning to look old.

"No way you're getting her, sir. She's all mine," Jacob said as he burst through the door. "Just kidding, of course. Just need to grab the old butterfly chair here and head back over to Ralph's. Nice to see you, sir," he added, sticking a hand out for dad.

"David, please, Jacob. Nice to see you, too," said Daddy. "I know she's in the retail clothing business for life. She's made that clear."

"Would you like a glass of wine, ah, David?" Jacob asked, rocking from foot to foot. Daddy clearly made him nervous.

"Yes, Daddy would love a glass, Jacob," I said while Jacob poured. "How's Ralph?"

"He's really down. Maybe this will help. I don't know," Jacob said, grabbing a new bottle, his corkscrew, and his butterfly chair and making a getaway.

"He's an interesting young man. I'm glad you have somebody to trust to run things until you get back," Daddy said. "I wish I had that."

"Good grief, Daddy. Ask Henry again. He loves his practice, and now that he's almost made partner, I don't know how he'd manage, especially with the kids and me," I said, "but ask him, OK?" Daddy liked Henry from the beginning. He always thought Alex was soft, wishy-washy, and spoiled. Old-money lazy. But Henry, son of an entrepreneur, understood the real world, Daddy liked to say.

"Would it be all right if I took Henry golfing, just for a long weekend?" Dad asked. "We'll head to Pennsylvania or South Carolina. Just so he and I could talk. I'd like his input on a few things, if nothing else."

"It's a great idea. He needs a break. Just don't pressure him too hard, OK? His family has dreams for him too," I said, knowing Daddy knew those realities, knowing he wished he had a son or, for that matter, a daughter interested in burgers.

"Is there anything you need, Jennifer? Anything at all?" he asked, walking around the room before stopping in front of the table between my two chairs. "That's the party invitation list, right?" He picked up the pages. "I still wish you'd rethink the whole thing. You're going to get better and, well…" Daddy said, his voice trailing off.

"It's a celebration about that, Daddy, promise. Anyway, Julie had an idea in case people are disappointed. When I get better, I'll refund people's travel expenses—sort of like a satisfaction guarantee," I said.

"I hate this entire conversation," he said, standing next to me and holding my hand, climbing back onto his pedestal. From on high he added, "I'm willing to support you in whatever you want to do. Promise me, though, after this party you will focus on something else?"

"Deal. And Daddy? I love you."

"I love you too, Jennifer," he said as he placed the pile of paper on my bedside table, kissed me on the top of my head, and self-consciously brushed nonexistent lint off the sleeve of his golf shirt as he walked out of the room.

"How'd it go?" Jacob asked, appearing in the door. He must've been hiding out there, waiting for the burger king's departure. "Ralph's asleep. Mind if I come in?"

The lonely, abandoned feeling was working its way up to my heart. The way I always felt when Daddy left. I was glad Jacob was there. "It went great. Let's get drunk and check the party list. I don't want to forget anybody from my past," I told him, forcing a smile as he plunked down the butterfly chair and shook it open.

"How will I know? I haven't known you all that long," he said.

"You know me as well as anyone, Jacob."

We both sat in silence, examining the names and addresses, catching typos. Jacob would sigh and shuffle papers around to let me know he was bored. But for me, the list represented the encounters of a lifetime. Everyone on it was a part of me. It was the ultimate Christmas card list. Except, unlike a Christmas card list, I'd be asking for more than a cursory greeting in return. I'd be asking for some time: a confrontation with mortality, a reflection.

Eventually Jacob coughed, jumped up, and grabbed the empty bottle of wine, our second, with Dad and Ralph's help. "Time to open another bottle and move on to something more interesting, I think. I mean, how many of these people do you expect, Jennifer?"

"I was hoping for ten from each decade of my life," I said.

"That's reasonable. Direct mail typically solicits a 2 percent response," Jacob said, sighing again, his boredom overtaking the last vestiges of his quick wit. It had been more than an hour of list reviewing and drinking.

"Let's avoid direct-mail comparisons shall we? I'm not sending them a coupon for laundry detergent," I said. "You're so weird sometimes."

"I'm reviewing an invitation list for a death party, and you think I'm weird?"

"Life celebration." I sighed, exasperated, and we both laughed.

6

Warning: Intentional misuse can be harmful.

MADDIE, SPORTING HER SIGNATURE ALL-BLACK ATTIRE, WHICH today included black leggings and an oversized black tee, was sitting cross-legged on my floor, like a pretzel, as they said in Hank's preschool class. Sitting next to Maddie in one of the chairs was Betsy, my trusted friend since elementary school. She looked exactly the same as she had in high school: brown hair, parted in the middle, stretching to the tops of her slender shoulders. We drank our first beer together, and made out with boys in her car, me with Alex and Betsy with his friend Paul. In the brown chair on the left Katie Sadler was Miss Prim and Proper with her blond bob, pink cardigan sweater, and legs crossed at her ankles. She wouldn't sit like a pretzel if her life depended on it. They were all part of my book club.

Since I hadn't been up to reading lately, my book club found other excuses for getting together. Great friends, all. Talented. Supportive. Stuffing envelopes in the name of the cause. Betsy and Katie were both married and lived near me in the suburban splendor of Grandville. Maddie lived with Lyle, her main squeeze, downtown in historic German Village. That's where Alex and I had both lived after college, and where we broke up, saying good-bye for good one fall night.

"I haven't been to a stuffing party since all your weddings and baby showers," Maddie said. "And I'm way ahead of all of you on my list. Look at this stack," she added proudly. "I've got to grab a smoke."

"OK, but you better be far away from the building. They're militant antismoking here," I said as Maddie headed for the green hall.

"I wish she'd get over that disgusting habit. It's going to kill her," Katie said and then looked up self-consciously at me. "Sorry."

"We're all going to die sometime. Some of us just get unlucky sooner," I said, with one of my regular responses formulated to ease others' discomfort. "Hey, how's Mister Right?"

"Great. We're going to Cabo San Lucas next weekend, sail fishing of all things. He rented a hacienda or something and, well, somebody should pinch me. I'm so happy," Katie said. The definition of elegant sophistication, she loved to wear simple sheath dresses. When she shopped at the Loop, she bought dresses that maximized her cleavage and her well-exercised body. She worked out at the gym five days a week and jogged on weekends. Her husband had been one of Grandville's most eligible bachelors before he met Katie. Gorgeous. Athletic. A dynamic and motivational speaker, Richie Sadler was the entrepreneurial spirit behind five restaurants in town. Not bad.

I wondered whether Katie's perfect life would suffer a twist of fate before I died. I had to admit, in my darkest times, I wished someone close to me would, just so I'd have a person to share my true feelings with. It was hard to be optimistic all the time.

I swallowed the bitterness that rose in my throat. They deserved their happiness. They didn't give me cancer.

"How many high school people did you invite, anyway? I mean, we had six hundred in our class. And those teachers?" Katie's face wrinkled in disgust. "Honestly, if I never thought about high school again, I'd be happy. It was a time to get through. I'm glad it's over."

"I only invited twenty from high school. No teachers, sadly enough," I said. "But I did invite Mrs. Murdock and Mrs. Purvis from fourth grade." I had to laugh at Betsy's rolling eyes. "Hey, they helped make us who we are today as much as friendship bracelets, you know".

"As long as you didn't invite Mrs. Belton. She was mean."

"Don't remind me. That woman never smiled. And don't worry. It's *my* party. I get to exercise selective memory on this one."

The phone interrupted our laughter. Katie answered it. It was Henry, checking to be sure I hadn't been drugged when I agreed to let him play golf, guilt-free, with Daddy. Actually, I felt pretty good. During rounds that morning, the doctors acted encouraged; apparently the immunotherapies were mobilizing my white blood cell counts—*Go, white team!* Even though it was the fourth quarter, the two-minute drill, the good guys were still in the game. Maybe they really could rally. Maybe the wine had helped?

"Are you sure, honey?" Henry had asked. "Your dad wants to be gone three nights. He said your mom and Julie would watch the kids—oh, and Julie's new nanny. Of course, Paige would still have them during the day. He wants to leave in the morning. As in, tomorrow."

"Great. I think you deserve it. I'll be fine. The kids will survive, I hope. I'll have Betsy check on them at Mother's this weekend," I said, looking over at Betsy, who nodded. "And your job is to forget about all of us and shoot a record round at Merion."

"How did you know?" he asked.

"A lucky guess. It's Daddy's favorite course, and his favorite showers," I said. "You have to go to Jim's and get a Philly cheesesteak with Cheese Whiz. Promise?"

"Promise. You're the best. I'll miss you," Henry said.

"You'll be staying at the Rittenhouse, on Rittenhouse Square. Be sure you stop in to the cute kids' store just up the street," I said.

"I'll call you tonight! Thanks again for the hall pass," Henry said, hanging up.

"Bye, love you," I managed, but he was gone. After hanging up the phone, I picked up a stack of envelopes and sorted through them while Katie regaled Betsy with a story about someone we all knew from high school. My college roommates, three favorite professors, four college boyfriends—I had taken advantage of the fact Alex and I went to separate schools, even if he hadn't.

Still, summers during college breaks were always spectacular, some of the best times of my life. I'd drive back into town and Alex would be waiting for me, wrapping me in a warm embrace filled with longing.

The months spent apart between Christmas and the end of the school year seemed the longest. And although he continued to swear off dating other girls during college, I didn't think it made sense. College—especially my Southern school—revolved around having dates, going to parties as a couple, as I had tried to explain to him. Even going to a football game required a date.

On one of these breaks, Alex had picked me up and driven me to our favorite picnic spot along the river. It had been our place since high school, and fortunately it still hadn't been discovered. "I've missed you terribly," Alex said.

"I've missed you too," I agreed. He was a great guy, probably my best friend.

Alex had taken care of everything, as usual, spreading out a picnic blanket, opening a bottle of chilled wine, and producing a chilled platter of shrimp.

"So, did you behave?" he asked, giving me a sideways look, a hint of anger and disappointment glinting in his dark eyes.

"Behave? I'm not a child, Alex," I answered, not enjoying this line of questioning but knowing it had been coming, as it did at the beginning of every summer. "School's out for the summer, and I cannot wait to spend it with you. When can we go to the lake house?"

Alex shook his head, as if chasing bad thoughts from his mind, thoughts of who I had dated in college this year, what I had done. Then he reached over and pulled my head down into his lap. "I don't know why I let you get away with everything, Jenn. I guess I just love you too much."

We made love on the blanket after the sunset, fireflies flittering around us. Alex wouldn't bring up any other men in my life until the end of the summer, I knew.

Now Maddie stepped back into the room. "You're not kidding about those militant bitches. They chased me to the end of the driveway," she said, settling back into her spot on my floor. "Hey, who's been messing with my piles?"

"Not messing, *organizing*," I said. "Told you they hated smoking."

When I looked up, Ralph was standing in my doorway, a big grin on his face.

"You look great! Come on in!" Whatever Jacob had said to him the night before, it worked.

"Hi, Jennifer. Hi, ladies," Ralph said, leaning against the door. "Barbara and I are going on a date tonight, to The Pearl, if you can believe it. We have reservations at seven thirty. Like regular people. My docs said it was fine."

"Ralph, I'm so happy for you," I said, although suddenly I was feeling like it would be a lonely weekend. The green monster was flaring up. I was accustomed to knowing Ralph would be there whenever I felt like talking. The Pearl was a four-star restaurant with a first-class hotel attached. I had a feeling he'd be gone as long as possible.

"You must try the scallops there," Katie said. "Last time Richie and I were there, they were to die—I mean, they were awesome."

"Sounds good," Ralph said, meeting eyes with me. "Jennifer and I are always looking for things to die for. See you," he added before disappearing.

"God, what is with me today? I'm sorry. This insensitivity bug seems to have bitten me pretty hard," Katie said, blushing. She seemed to think this was a new affliction.

I decided not to respond. "What's new in the wonderful world of gossip, Maddie?" I asked. "Any hot scandals?"

"Unfortunately, it's a little quiet these days. Football's starting up, back to school and all, and that keeps the wandering eyes close to home. For the time being. They get restless again come mid-September."

"And how's Lyle?" Katie asked.

"Well, I don't think he's going to whisk me away to a tropical island and propose anytime soon, if that's what you mean," Maddie answered. "It's just not his style." Lyle was a copywriter in an advertising agency. A sensitive guy. A nice guy. Probably one of the most normal struggling artists Maddie had dated so far.

"And John?" Katie asked, directing her prying attention to Betsy's husband.

"We're fine," Betsy chimed in. "We're ready to start trying for number two."

"There goes book club. More breast-feeding than reading," Maddie sniffed.

"Why don't you just tell us the exact moment and all the details of conception?" Katie said. "I just don't see why everybody tells everything about all that baby stuff these days. It's embarrassing. I know who's trying to get pregnant, who's taking their temperature, who's on fertility treatments. It's really all too personal."

"You'll be in the same boat, Katie, don't forget," I interjected before she could totally deflate Betsy. "For someone about to go on a tropical vacation, you're awfully negative."

"Sorry," she said. "You know, I've got to run. I told my boss I was at a luncheon meeting, but she'll know after three hours even the Public Relations Society of America would be over by now."

"I don't know. They seemed to go on forever when I was a member," I told her. "Man, I hated those. Unless you were on a committee, all the bigwigs ignored you. Besides, my primary focus then was trying to get Milton's mug in the news."

"By the way, Milton says hi," Katie told me, rolling her eyes. Milton was on everyone's unpopular list.

"Does Milton still suck up to you?" I asked Katie.

"Is the carpet always green at Shady Valley?" she answered, standing up and bringing me the few cards she hadn't stuffed. "Are you up to finishing my pile?"

"Sure. And thanks for coming, Katie. It means a lot," I said.

"No problem. And remember, next month's book is *The Red Badge of Courage*—do you need it on tape?" Katie asked.

"I read it in school twice, but I'll let you know," I answered, watching Katie's tiny-heeled shoes tap across the floor. I had spotted the name Liza McBride at the top of Katie's pile. The "it" girl in high school. She symbolized everything I thought I wanted to be back then. I wondered as I stuffed her invitation if she was happy. Did she ever wonder about me?

I could still call to mind vivid memories of her. At our winter dance, eighth grade, a slow dance song cleared the floor, and everything but Liza and her boyfriend, the cutest boy in school, seemed to stop. We all stared at them in the center of the room. That was my first glimpse of romantic love, beyond the movies—in person. And it was amazing. They stared into each other's eyes, Liza in a long blue dress that glittered and complemented her long blond hair. I can still taste the punch I was drinking as we watched, all of us girls who'd come as a group, huddled together, trying not to appear overtly jealous. And failing. It wasn't until I met Alex that I understood what Liza felt like.

Alex and I met at a party, much like any other high school party. Ginny's parents were out of town, and several of us were spending the night. Word spread, and suddenly more than a hundred kids from school had swarmed her house. I hadn't really talked to Alex before, but he seemed mysterious, floating around the outskirts of the crowd. I was shy too, so the likelihood of our talking was low, until we found ourselves pushed into the same corner of Ginny's living room.

"This is going to get rolled by the cops," he said, taking a sip from his Heineken. Expensive, aloof, mysterious.

"Probably," I agreed, taking a sip from my Miller Lite. Inexpensive, bland, and, well, common.

"Want to go outside? We can sit in my car. It's just around the corner."

Looking around, I couldn't find Ginny, or any of the other girls I was spending the night with. The room felt as if it would explode from the sheer mass of kids, and I did want to get out of there. "Sure," I answered, and that was the start of a long and mostly wonderful relationship. Before he dropped me off at my house we talked for hours, about life and high school, dreams, and our families. It was as if we'd always been friends. We agreed on so much. We were the perfect pair.

An hour later, Betsy and Maddie gathered the invites to drop off at the post office. We had sorted the out-of-state cards; they needed to go overnight. The rest, the in-town cards, would just be delivered first-class mail. Everybody had about two weeks to plan on attending or to blow me off. What if nobody came? Did that mean my life wasn't significant? Or did it just confirm everybody's worst fear: in the end, all you have is yourself? Yourself and your memories.

It was too late now. Maddie and Betsy were gone. Juliana had given her blessing. Like an out-of-control freight train, my farewell party was underway.

So I called Jacob, but the machine at the Loop picked up. Eerie that my voice on the recording would last longer than my voice in real life. *I need to shake out of this morbidity.* It was strange and hard to describe, these feelings that came pulsing at me from deep inside, from the cancer—deep sorrow, joy, moments of terror, but also moments of peace, and also purpose, the desire to live in the moment. To hold a party and see the important people in my life. I should be happy for Ralph. He was off to enjoy a gourmet-restaurant date with his wife at a place famous for candlelight, fine cuisine, and old-fashioned romance.

I enjoyed a gourmet meal for the first time with Alex. Because of Mother's California roots, we ate healthy, lots of vegetables and fruits and all. But we didn't eat fancy, not until later, when Mother acquired her first chef. Before that, we ate meatloaf and spaghetti and the regular all-American stuff. Alex's old-money family always enjoyed the best of everything, including food.

Alex was born with a shiny silver spoon firmly held in his perfect mouth. My first car was a brown Ford Mustang. His first car was a silver Jaguar. My dad believed that children should work as soon as they turned sixteen, and work hard, just not at the family business. He got me my first summer job, as a cashier at Target. Yippee. Meanwhile, Alex, like he had every summer, hung out at the country club pool, swimming and playing an occasional game of tennis.

Looking back, I had to smile at my teenage angst. Working at Target probably taught me more about the retail market than all my years of college, but at the time it seemed like pure torture.

Alex drove me to work my first day. I was wearing the red shirt, dreading meeting my fellow cashiers. They'd know I wasn't from around there. At least I had the sense to know they shouldn't see my boyfriend's car. I told him to drop me off at the far corner of the shopping center parking lot. No matter what, he wasn't ever to come inside or pull up in front driving that car. When that day finally ended, I clocked out and, like a spy, ran through the parking lot, glancing over my shoulder to be sure no one was watching. Spotting Alex, I grinned. He'd wedged his Jag in between a red pickup truck and a 7UP delivery truck.

"So, how's my favorite cashier?" Alex asked, leaning over to kiss me. "Umm, you smell so, well, corn doggish. Kind of like that state-fair smell, you know?"

"Great. Thanks," I pouted. "I can't do this all summer. This isn't building character like Daddy says—this is stupid."

"Finished?" Alex asked as we sped down Morse Road. I glared at him. "Good. Open this," he said, handing me a blue box tied with a white satin bow. Tiffany's. It was a diamond solitaire necklace. It sparkled in the fading sunlight.

He drove to the river, and as the sun began to droop, Alex set up a picnic in the place that would become our spot. A picnic of iced shrimp, brie, chilled champagne. A world away from Target. At sixteen, I thought his world seemed like a dream world, and I wanted to be a part of it forever.

Suddenly, I was aware my dinner tray had arrived on my bedside table. The meal didn't look any better than lunch. I wasn't the least bit hungry. I wondered if I ever would be again. I wondered if I could stomach a gourmet meal if it magically appeared. Instead of eating, I decided to sleep.

Alex said, "Remember all those times we drove to the river and watched the sunset? We should do that again. Let's do it now."

"*The best part about it was how you took the time to be romantic. I feel like since I turned thirty, everything has been rushed.*"

"*But you* are *happy, aren't you?*" *Alex asked, spreading out the red-and-white-checked picnic blanket.*

"*I hope so.*"

"*Let's have a toast, then. To us and the future,*" *Alex said.*

"*Cheers. I'll just have a sip,*" *I said, raising my glass to meet his and watching the legs of the wine along the side of the glass, the light from the citronella candle on the tablecloth adding to the calm as the sun sunk into the brown water of the river.*

He leaned over and kissed me on the lips, softly at first, more passionately as I found myself returning the kiss eagerly, hungrily. We were rolling across the blanket and he was pressing against me. "Wait, Alex, we're going too fast."

"*Are you kidding? I've been waiting years, Jennifer—*"

"Jennifer, wake up. You're dreaming," a voice that sounded just like Alex's said.

"I'm up, I'm up," I said, waking with a start to find myself almost nose to nose with Alex, the perpetrator of my dreams. Did he know? My pillow was wet with drool. What had I said? Was I flushed?

"Your sister told me Henry went golfing with your dad, so I thought you might like some company," Alex said, leaning in as I tried to sit up. We bumped foreheads. I smiled and blushed.

"Alex, could you give me a couple of minutes?" I said.

"Sure. I hope you're hungry, because I brought a picnic of all your favorites. I'll just take this good old tray of nondescript food items out to those friendly, helpful nurses and give you some time alone," Alex said, smoothing out the covers before grabbing the tray of food I'd ignored earlier.

"It is all right if I stay, isn't it?" he asked, poking his head back in the door.

"I'd love it," I answered. *Where are Stripes or Nurse Mary Ann when I need them? Heck, even Hadley would do.* I hated to use it, but the walker in the corner was a necessity when primping time wasn't plentiful, so I shuffled over to it in all its stainless-steel glory. By the time I finished, emerging after a quick shower, my room was transformed. The curtains were drawn, and the lights were dimmed to barely a glow. In the middle of the floor was a candlelight picnic on a red-and-white-checkered cloth just like in my dream. I swallowed—hard.

"Welcome to Romeo's Ristorante," Alex said. "Allow me to show you to your seat." Once I settled into a beanbag chair Alex had brought, I had a chance to look around. I was glad I'd taken my pain medication and had a pain lollipop in my pocket, just in case.

"Alex, you're too much." I watched him pour red wine into crystal glasses. Was I supposed to be having a picnic with the man I almost married? Why not? This was what I had in mind for my going-away party. Most people wouldn't bring me a picnic, though.

"I doubt your dad would've taken me away for a golf weekend if we'd gotten married," Alex said, handing me the glass of wine. He was right. "Oysters on the half shell?" I almost choked on my wine. I didn't trust myself to share my nocturnal fantasy with Alex without blushing, so I simply nodded and smiled. Besides, given the circumstances, it still felt oddly real.

"Daddy's more sophisticated than that," I said defensively, adding, "You're right, though—he thought you were a wimp and that I could do better."

"At least his dreams came true. Cheers!" Alex said a little too brightly.

"Mothers always liked you," I said, suddenly wanting him to know she did. "She was crushed when we broke up for good."

Speaking of good…this food was amazing. I guess I had my answer about my appetite. I could still eat. I smiled at Alex and sliced a piece of brie. It was soft, just gooey enough to be perfect on the crackers Alex had brought. The candlelight flickered and danced around the striped walls of my room. The glow was warm, and different. So much different than what I'd grown accustomed to in here. I needed more candles, more seafood, more cheese in my life, I decided.

"Man, did I pine away for you during school. Sometimes I thought I wouldn't make it. Look at this," he said, rummaging around in the big wicker picnic basket. He handed me a photograph. "Remember this?"

I looked at our smiling faces in the photo. So young and full of ourselves and our shared adventure. We had everything then and not a clue as to what the world had in store for us.

"There we are on the train, from Luxembourg to Bruges. Not many college kids spend Thanksgiving in Europe with their boyfriend," I said, indulging his ego. We had had so many fun times together.

"If only you hadn't called me Chuck in bed, it would've been perfect," Alex teased.

I threw a shrimp at him. I didn't want him to turn the mood to serious or dark. I needed light, I needed a friend, and we'd been over all this, years ago. "Look, that was nearly fifteen years ago now, for heaven's sake. You've been married and divorced."

"Yeah, and I dreamed you would be too," Alex said, leaning over toward me, placing the meaty part of the shrimp in my mouth. "Bite." His lips were smiling, but his eyes weren't. His look was serious.

Yikes, I thought. Did I feel the same? No, I was happy, with Henry, with our life. "Bite me," I replied sarcastically, hoping to lighten the mood. His dark eyes were inches from mine, and I knew he was waiting for the slightest signal that I wanted more. This was surreal. *Am I still asleep?*

"My pleasure, Jenn. You always did like it a little on the rough side, as I recall. Remember that huge bathtub in Paris? We made love so many times I didn't think you would walk again."

I felt my face flush with the memory. I took a long sip of wine and stared at the photo, willing my heart to beat at a normal pace. It had been ages since anyone had talked to me about making love. When Henry first swept me off my feet, he only had to wink at me to make my knees weak. If he said the word "sex," well, we had to have it. *How long ago was that? Is it gone forever for us?*

"Look, Alex," I said, settling back a bit on my beanbag chair. "You're making me uncomfortable. We had such great times together. We were best friends. But that was in the past."

"We were more than best friends. One more from memory lane," Alex said, handing me a photo of us at his senior year fraternity formal.

"Until that party, all the other guys thought you were my imaginary friend. You didn't come to one party in four years of college. Finally you showed up, wild hair and all, and wowed 'em," Alex said, his dark brown eyes glistening in the flickering candlelight.

In the picture, Alex smiled broadly, his hair slicked back and his tuxedo perfectly pressed. I was wearing a navy dress with a high, rounded neck and cap sleeves. My ears sparkled with the diamond studs he had given me during our second week in Europe. We were holding hands. It had been a wonderful weekend.

"I remember that weekend was so much fun, meeting all your friends," I said quietly. I knew I had hurt Alex throughout our relationship by not being as fully committed as he was. I hoped we could get past this—this past hurt—and move on to something, here, now, friends once more.

Alex put the photos away and pushed the wicker basket to the corner of the blanket. He leaned onto the beanbag chair, his breath tickling my cheek. The softness was back in his eyes. "Are you comfortable?" he asked. "Do you hurt a lot?"

"The pain isn't bad tonight, Alex, thanks," I said, and it was true. I hadn't even touched the lollipop in my pocket. "This picnic was such a wonderful surprise."

"Well, I'm not leaving yet—I'm just checking. And speaking of checking, when do the drill sergeants check in on you?" he asked.

"Usually around ten. But I can flip a switch, and it lights up a "do not disturb" sign in the hall, and supposedly they won't come in unless I call them," I explained. "They can leave my medicine in the pass-through." *Why am I telling him that? What am I doing?*

"Great. Where's the switch?" Alex asked, jumping up.

"By my throne—I mean, bed," I answered, watching him move gracefully to the bedside and flip the switch. Alex was fluid, not squared and defined like Henry. More graceful. Royal boy versus beach boy. Panther versus lion.

"A throne fit for my queen. Remember when I proposed, Jennifer?" he asked, sitting back down next to me on the beanbag chair. Our arms were touching from elbow to shoulder. I got a chill. We didn't need to go down this road again, not now. Not when our time together had been so special tonight. Not now.

"It was beautiful, Alex, really."

"Yeah, so beautiful you said no," he said, his jaw tightening at the memory.

"I didn't turn you down-down, Alex," I said, looking at my wedding ring—the one from Henry. "I said 'yes, but not yet.'"

"Oh, you were a perfect diplomat, Jennifer, and clever. So very clever at covering your bases," Alex said with unmistakable bitterness. Bitterness that had simmered for many years. "If you had said yes, then, well…" He blew out the candle then. His lips—I remembered those sweet, soft lips—brushed gently across mine. I wanted to make it up to him somehow. To erase the bitterness with the passion that still swelled at the sight of him. I wanted him. For then. For now. Forever. To make me well with the wanting. I needed to feel this again, to feel this alive. *And I can feel this. I'm still in here, still me.* Where had this feeling gone? *Henry has been here by my side, but not here, like this, not since I got sick. Where did he go? Where did Alex go? My god.*

"I didn't think we'd ever lose each other," I said, and then adding, dangerously, "I didn't want to lose you."

Alex looked away for a long time as we sat in the silent darkness. At last, he wrapped his arms around me and pulled me onto his lap.

"Oh, my baby, you're so thin," he whispered. "I really wanted to take care of you. I can't bear losing you again."

"This isn't happening, is it?" I asked, feeling trapped somewhere between my dreams of how life should be and how it was. Somewhere between the truth—and the make-believe.

"Just for tonight, pretend we never were lost," Alex whispered as his hand began gently caressing my chest. "Does this hurt, my holding you?"

"No," I said, feeling his warm breath on my neck. "Alex, no," I said now, meaning it and not. It was enough for me that he wanted me as much as I wanted him. I wasn't ready to take it further, even if in my mind I already had.

"I won't do anything you don't want me to do, Jennifer. Just relax," he said. He picked me up and carried me to my bed, crawling in next to me. His right arm cradled my neck as his right hand brushed my cheek. I allowed myself to drift off in the safety of his embrace, while my body accepted his gentle caresses.

I awoke with a start and a sharp pang of guilt.

"Alex, I loved having you here tonight, but I think you need to go," I whispered, not sure if he was awake or asleep behind me. I couldn't pretend any longer. My life was with Henry.

When I turned, I found Alex staring up at the ceiling. His fingers found my arm, caressed it. I turned my head, heard him turn his, and felt his breath on my hair. "OK, but can I see you again tomorrow?" he asked. "Jennifer?"

"Sure," I answered finally, feeling him get out of bed. I turned to watch him. "Yes, please."

"Can I kiss you good night?" he asked, once the picnic was tucked back into the basket.

I didn't answer. He walked over to the throne again anyway.

"Sweet dreams, princess," he said, kissing me once more on the lips. Slowly. Sweetly.

7

Warning: Close cover before striking.

I WAS WATCHING THE NEWS, HEARING ABOUT ANOTHER TRAFFIC fatality, wondering who the person was who died, old or young, at fault or innocent. How would he or she be remembered? How would I?

If I didn't make it (that nasty, looming *if*), Hannah would consider me as The Perfect Mom. Think about it. I'd never scolded her, grounded her, stuck her in time out. I'd be an image on the wall, a figure floating over her in her dreams, an inaccessible link to her past. A weight over her future. Unmoving, unchanging, unaging. Untouchable.

For Hank, I'd be a bit more real. But still weak, reclining. Still a doll. I hoped he would remember my laugh. I inherited it from my great-aunt on my father's side: a hearty, robust, conversation-stopping laugh—not very perfect, unfortunately, but very real. That's why I'd been making videos and writing about myself. I wanted to be more than a flat memory to my kids. It had taken me a while to get the hang of it, but by now I had stockpiled about an hour's worth of footage.

The first time, as soon as the red light of the camera turned on, I froze. The camera was new but just like the one we'd bought before Hank was born, so I knew how to use it to video other people. When I turned the stupid lens on myself for the first time, I choked. I opened my mouth, and nothing came out.

I'd read on a survivor's blog about how to leave a lasting legacy for your kids, and one of the writer's ideas was this—a video series. That was six months after my diagnosis, before I came to Shady Valley. I had finished surgery and chemo. Wearing makeup and a hat, I tried to look my best. I sat in the bedroom I still shared with Henry on our small yellow couch by our bay window. I propped the camera on our coffee table on top of a stack of books. The kids were napping, I locked the door so Paige couldn't come in—and I froze.

Take two. "Hi kids, it's Mommy, and I wanted to tell you a little about me and how much I love you," I managed to say before the tears started. I gave myself a pep talk and started again.

Take three. "There really is nothing more amazing than being a mom. It's such a gift. Such a responsibility. I hope you know that even though I haven't been able to be right there with you, all the time, I've been with you in my heart. And I will be. Always."

During quiet moments, when I wasn't distracted by visitors or nurses or tests, my thoughts drifted to my kids' elementary school years.

"What was your real mommy like?" Hannah's friends will ask quietly, so they won't upset Henry's new young wife stirring mac and cheese at my kitchen counter. *She'll be thin, work out every day, and she'll be a model. No, an attorney. An attorney who does modeling on the side. She'll want to have two kids too, so she will be even with me. Only I know she never will be, because I'll be timeless.*

Perfect. Henry will comfort her by telling her that I had become simply a problem he couldn't fix. An irregular occurrence for a man accustomed to solving anything life threw his way. He was one of the lucky ones, the 1 percent. A go-to guy. Have a question? Here's the answer. Except for my cancer—in the face of this, this all-encompassing, cell-mutating thing, he was helpless. They would hug and be glad they had each other and their perfect life together, even if a few wrinkles appeared along the way. I would be the weight of the past; she will be the light of the future.

"No," I said aloud. I needed to be in the future. I needed to hold out a few more years. I'd call my doctor, see if anything new had come around. If I could last five years, that would be like fifty years to Hank and Hannah. Kid time moved so slowly. I remembered how long it took to get to Christmas from Thanksgiving when I was little. I could make it to elementary school, even to middle school surely.

Later that afternoon, Betsy poked her brunette head in my doorway. She hadn't started to show yet, but she did have the pregnancy glow I noticed now. Her bright-yellow sundress flowed freely. She looked so happy, so fulfilled. The dimples punctuating her cheeks always made me smile. As with anyone I knew and cared about who was pregnant, I worried about genes malfunctioning. What if she became another me?

"Why so gloomy today, Jennifer? Missing Henry?" Betsy asked, the dimples disappearing as concern crossed her face. She tucked her hair behind her ears, her nervous habit. She said she had come by to report that all the invitations were mailed, but I was willing to bet Henry told her to check on me.

"I dunno," I huffed. *What a grump.* "I'm sorry, Betsy. Just bored, I guess.

"It's OK to be gloomy—I understand."

No, I thought, *you couldn't possibly understand.* What if I told the truth? Confessed that I was jealous of Ralph and his wife and their romantic date together? Ticked that I let Henry and Daddy go golfing, even for a few days? Mad that I didn't make love to Alex last night? Depressed about Henry's future without me, with his new and unbelievably perfect wife? Would she really understand after all?

"Alex is back in town. He came here, last night, with a picnic," I said. Betsy didn't look surprised at the news. *She knew he was in town. She knew.*

"You know, Jennifer, he always was great at that romantic kind of stuff. But you were never really happy with him. He gave you too much freedom, and you took it. You didn't respect him, really. Henry is so much better for you, much more your equal. And Alex, well, I don't know if he's necessarily the same sweet guy you remember," Betsy said as she re-tucked her brown hair back behind each of her ears. She wore chic, camel-color flats that I bet were from the Loop. Her toes were painted a perky pink. "I mean, it's been a long time."

"I realize that. I'm not interested in a relationship, for God's sake. I just said he came by, that's all," I snapped. I couldn't look at her, and I knew I sounded defensive. In the old days, Betsy had always stood up for Alex, so I was caught off guard by her tone. Why was she picking on the only person who was making me feel alive? Didn't she know I needed him right now?

"Hey, don't get mad. I'm trying to help. What do you want from him? What does he want from you? I thought that part of your life was over. Can you two really just be friends? It always ended in disaster before," she said, climbing up on the throne, yellow sundress flowing around her. "You'd break up, he'd whine to me, to your sister, even to your mom. You'd start another relationship, with some other guy, and the minute things hit a rough spot, you'd be running back to Alex. And he'd take you back."

"His choice," I noted stubbornly.

"Not normal," she said. "We all were relieved when it was finally over, and he'd moved on. Don't play with fire, Jenn."

"Really, Betsy? Look at me. I'm not playing with fire; I'm not playing with anything. I'm fighting for my life, and I'll take all the companionship friends have to offer," I said, folding my arms across my chest.

Betsy just stared.

"Look, I don't know. I don't. Can you go back to friends after you've been so much more for so long?" I asked.

"If you're determined to find out, then you've got the weekend to do that without upsetting Henry. But I'd be careful, Jennifer. That's all I'm saying," she said. Somehow, her hands had found her hips in the sea of yellow, and she wasn't showing either dimple. She was serious, staring into my eyes. I looked down at my hands. "Don't hurt Alex again. Don't hurt Henry. And most of all, don't complicate things, Jenn. Look at you—you don't need more complications."

"Betsy, I know, and that's not what I'm doing. I just get lonely, and no one is here, and no one can understand. Not you. Not anyone," I said. I looked down at my hands, knowing I was wrong, wanting to be right. I felt so alone. "I'm not complicated, Bets. I'm alone."

"No, you're not. I'm here. Henry's here—he's just golfing. Your kids and your mom and dad are here. You have everything—more than most people. Stop trying to mess things up," Betsy said, tears in her eyes. "I don't trust Alex. I don't trust you with Alex. I think it's a bad idea for you to see him.

"Mommmmeeeee," Hank screeched, bursting into the room at just the right time. I'd had enough advice.

Betsy stood and watched the scene, tears, damning tears, rolling down her cheeks.

"Hi, my little cherub," I told Hank, ignoring Betsy and turning onto my side, hoisting Hank up next to me on the throne. This would last about a second. Yep.

"I wanna get down now. Play," he said, arching his back to get out of our hug.

I looked over at Betsy. "In the end, we're all alone, Bets," I said. "But thank you for trying, for helping. I love you."

"I love you too," Betsy said, and walked out the door.

Paige arrived a good minute after Hank had barreled in, carried Hannah to me, and placed her on top of my chest, in my arms. She grinned at me.

"She's so beautiful," I said to no one as she babbled and began to push away, ready to cruise. I wanted to hold her as a little girl. I didn't want to be The Perfect Mom in her dreams. But, as usual, she was crawling away from me.

The next morning, I was watching the news again when my telephone rang. It was Juliana. I put her on speakerphone and muted the TV.

"Jennifer, it's so hard to plan a 'progressive' menu," she whined through the speaker. "I just don't understand what you want me to do. And how am I supposed to make that, that *institution* have any ambiance for a party, for heaven's sake? It would be so much nicer at our home, don't you think?" She added, "And the replies, they're just pouring in. I practically need a secretary to keep up with the scheduling. It's just not working."

"Mother, calm down," I told her, trying to focus on her groaning while the roar in my head grew louder. The dam of calm was about to break. "The whole point was supposed to be for me to spend time with people I care about, OK? The food, the ambiance, the time—none of that is really that important, OK?" Yes, I was now the spoiled brat.

"Fine," Mother said, sounding pouty.

"Mother, you're great at this stuff. I know whatever you do will be just perfect, and, Mother, I really do appreciate all your trouble."

"Oh my. Oh, I must run," Juliana said, making a sucking kissing sound into the telephone before hanging up. I was glad I'd had her on speakerphone. That sucking kiss creeped me out.

Ralph knocked and poked his head in. "Thanks for the official invitation, Jennifer," he said. "They turned out really nice, yes siree."

"Come in. Tell me about your fantastically romantic evening, as long as you get rid of the fake cowboy crap," I said. I was beginning to get over my jealousy and was genuinely happy for my best friend.

He shuffled in, grinning from ear to ear. An idiot cowboy.

"You know, the food there is 'to die for,'" he said, and we both laughed as he settled into the right brown chair.

"So, was it as good as going to the wine country?" I asked.

"Better," he said. "We finally talked. All this time, at least the past six months, we've been going through the motions. She's been trying to hold things together at home while I've been focused on trying to live. Doing these stupid treatments, feeling worse instead of better."

"But that's all you can do, that's all *we* can do, here," I said, waving my hand to encompass this space, my room, us, Shady Valley.

"No, it's not all we can do, Jenn," Ralph said quietly. "We need to appreciate all they are doing to support us. We need to tell them thank you more, at least I do. You're probably better at this with Henry and your people than I am, but I haven't told Barbara thank you in so long. 'Thank you for taking care of our family so I can take care of my health, Barb. I am so lucky to have you, and I love you.' That's what she needed to hear; it's what I needed to say, what I should have been saying. We had a great meal, a great talk, and then we actually made love. It was the best night of my life."

Ralph paused. He had been looking out the window as he was talking. Tears were streaming down my face as we sat there in silence.

"I'm so happy for you, for both of you. And you're right, of course," I finally said. "I used to text Henry all the time, call him too, and tell him I loved him. I don't do that anymore. I never do that anymore." I wondered when I had stopped.

My telephone was ringing. "It might be Henry. I better answer it," I said, looking apologetically at Ralph, who shrugged. It was Henry.

"I am having the best time. I love Philly, your dad. Thank you so much for letting me come—I love it," he added.

"Wow, that's a lot of love," I said sarcastically. Ralph mouthed, "Thank you." He wanted me to tell Henry thank you, but I wasn't feeling it, even though it wasn't Henry's fault that he was there and Alex was here and I was dying.

"We're going to a restaurant in the Italian Market district tonight. Tony's or something. Your dad loves it," Henry was saying.

"Mmm-hmmm," I said, rolling my eyes at Ralph. And Ralph mouthed, "Be nice." I rolled my eyes again. "Henry needs a break too," Ralph whispered.

"And I went to Born Yesterday," Henry said, "that kid's store, and I went crazy buying stuff for Hannah. Hank too, of course, but girls' clothes are so cute. Did you know, at Merion, where we played, the top of the flag sticks are woven baskets? No flags."

"Amazing. I'm so glad you're having fun, Henry," I tried. Ralph nodded approval. Henry was really too happy to be talking to me right then. "Are you the burger prince yet?"

"Your dad's mentioned the idea briefly. He knows how I feel about my practice. I've worked so hard. We'd need to work things out. But it's pretty intriguing." He paused. "Enough about me. How are you feeling?"

"Fine. Tired. The kids were here with Paige. Mother called. I think my party's starting to stress her out. But it sounds like a lot of people are responding. That'll be fun," I said.

"I'd enjoy it if some old girlfriends showed up—not just all old boyfriends," he teased.

I dropped my voice and turned away from Ralph. "Oh Henry, really. What does it matter? I'm yours now, for the rest of my life. Not much of a deal, but it's all I've got. I guess you could be scouting my replacement," I said, writhing in self-pity. "You've got to be sick of this, this sickness. And if you are, I'd understand. You really should start looking around. A young female attorney at the firm, perhaps?"

"You sound awful. Do you want me to come home?" Henry asked.

Yes. You should come home, I thought. *Come home and be with me because there are other guys who want to be with me, who find me attractive still, even like this, and that's nice.*

"No. I'm fine. Like I said, just a little tired. Ralph's here. He'll cheer me up," I told him, glancing over at Ralph, who put his pointer fingers at the corners of his mouth, willing me to smile. It didn't work.

"I love you, Jennifer. I'll be home Tuesday evening, and I'll come straight there," Henry said before hanging up.

I looked down at the dead receiver in my hand. *He should hop on a plane. He should do it now. I told him how I was feeling. Why doesn't he get it? Why doesn't he see I really need him? I need him now, before we lose everything.*

Ralph said, "I'll let you get some rest, Jennifer, but before I go I just want to thank you. For the wine. For the encouragement. For sending Jacob over. Barbara just needed to vent—and really, it was good for both of us. Just a small break, but last night it felt like we were newlyweds again. Maybe it'll be the same for you and Henry. Maybe that's what you both need too."

"Or maybe I just need sex," I said. "Sorry. I'm Oscar tonight. You should paint me green and stick me in a trash can."

"We all feel like that sometimes, even you. Go to sleep, Jennifer. It's eight o'clock, a perfectly acceptable bedtime," Ralph said, kissing me platonically on the head as he prepared to make his escape. "You're going to be OK, kid. Give Henry a chance. They are suffering too."

"I know. But it doesn't seem like it when he's playing golf at one of the best courses in the world, and I'm here. Is he suffering, really?" I asked. Ralph didn't answer but pulled my door shut tight.

Eight o'clock. Why wasn't Alex here? Where was he? Why hadn't he called? Why did I care?

I called Jacob. I knew I'd get his voice mail. As soon as it beeped, I blurted out a message: "Juliana is going crazy because the party is too much for her. People are coming out of the woodwork. This is a good thing, isn't it? Doesn't it mean they care? Shouldn't she be glad? I need your help setting up a sitting area here, and maybe a bar, and, well, whatever you think. You don't need to call me back tonight—I know you and Nelson always have a date on Saturday nights. By the way, is it possible to love two people enough to be married to both of them? Even if you're not Mormon? Is it wrong to want it all before it's all too late? Let me know. Good night."

Night. I was going to spend this Saturday night alone, I guess. *That's OK.* I could watch the latest news. *No, I can't. Not tonight.* Tears were streaming down my face, blurring my eyesight. *I should just die. That would be the honorable, the best, outcome. No more suffering, no more living in the past. Henry would be happy: the kids could have a normal life with the new Mrs. Benson. Mother could plan a big funeral service, and Daddy, well, he'd have Henry, his heir apparent.* Nobody needed me; nobody could relate to me. Not really. Not ever again. I was too tired to try anymore.

The little blonde girl was standing with her back to me, hands on her hips, floating on a cloud, out of reach. A little cloud girl, taunting me: "I want to know who my daddy is, is that too much to ask?"

"Why do you have a Southern accent?" I asked the cloud girl, floating, as I was, on my own cloud.

"Is that relevant?" she demanded.

What a brat. *"It's my dream, isn't it?"*

"That depends."

I'm arguing with myself, *I thought, but then I realized the little brat was Julie.*

"Jennifer, wake up," Julie's voice said. The voice smelled like a very dry martini, extra olives. I woke up. It was her, minus the cloud and with a face. A very "done" face. I'd say at least a two-hour makeup job.

"Julie, what are you doing here? What time is it?" I asked, rolling over, trying to focus on the clock.

"It's only nine thirty, but we'll leave if you'd like," she said.

I saw him standing behind her. Alex? I was stunned and angry.

"We just had the most fabulous dinner. Mother asked Claire to come in special," Julie said. "And, of course, we invited Alex over, since he was all alone. He's in the same boat as little ol' me."

Why was Alex at dinner with Julie at my parents' house when he said he'd be here with me? I just blinked my swollen-from-crying eyes at the two of them.

"Jennifer, we should've called, made sure you were up to visitors. I told Julie I was planning a visit tonight, and somehow time got away from me, and the next thing you know, it was late," Alex said, still standing partially behind Julie. I could see half of a navy-blue summer sports coat, half of a white button-down, shirt and half of a smile.

"Time flies, you know, when you're having fun," I said, forcing myself to act calm. I wanted to cry, or better yet, go back to sleep and forget this entire day. It really couldn't get any worse.

"Well, I think little Jennifer needs some rest, don't you?" Julie said in her best Pollyanna imitation, slipping her arm through his. "We can visit some other time." She pulled on his arm while I watched. I wished I had Hadley's hammer.

"Excuse me, Julie, can I have a minute with Jennifer, alone?" Alex asked, finally stepping around my sister and taking my hand. I yanked it away.

"Well, whatever," Julie said, turning, wobbling away from my bed. I heard her drop into one of the brown chairs, imitating the spoiled cloud-child in my dream.

"I'm sorry. I should've called. Dinner lasted forever. I had too much wine. Will you forgive me?" he asked, bending his head close to mine, his soft lips so close. *No*, I told myself and crossed my arms over my chest.

Finally I asked, "Forgive you for being late or for being late because you had a long dinner with Julie?" I was glad Ralph had dimmed the lights because my swollen eyelids were making it hard enough to see.

"For both, I guess."

"I guess that depends," I whispered, aware of Julie straining to hear not five feet away.

"On what?" he asked softly.

"Why don't you come back tomorrow and we can talk about it. Alone." I squeezed my eyes closed, and Alex squeezed my shoulder. I didn't know what I wanted anymore. But I did know I'd had enough of this day.

"Good night, love," Alex whispered to me before escorting my sister from the room, his hand on the small of her back.

I shuddered at his intimacy, with me and with Julie. It was wrong. I knew it. Enough, again. Alex and my sister were cut from the same cloth. They should be together. I have a family. I am whole. Wholly sad, but whole.

8

Warning: Not suitable for all audiences.

"Good morning, sunshine," Alex said, waltzing into my room carrying a huge bouquet of roses he placed on my bedside table. He was dressed in what can only be described as Italian stud clothing—fitted dress pants, white shirt. His presumptuous attitude honked me off, but I was intrigued he was here.

"What do you want, Alex?" I asked, covering my morning breath with my hand.

"Want? Well, you, of course," he said. "How did you sleep?"

Really, what was this? Last night he'd arrived late, with my sister, drunk. Now he was bringing flowers and waltzing into my room like he owned it, owned me. "Alex, what are you doing here? Why were you eating with Julie and my parents last night? What's going on? Is it some sort of weird revenge?"

"Revenge? Love of my life, you need some coffee," Alex said and, as usual, produced what I needed, in this case, a cup of coffee nestled inside a basket I hadn't seen until now. "Black, French, perfect temperature."

"Thanks," I said. At least the coffee would cover up my morning breath, and I knew Nurse Hadley would come to the rescue soon.

She always did. I took a heavenly sip and asked the question that had been on the top of my mind since last night: "So, how much time have you and Julie been spending together?"

Alex choked on his coffee, confirming what I thought and had decided in my rational, nonhormone-driven dreams last night. Julie and Alex belonged together. And that was fine. Henry and I belonged together, and that was perfect.

As he walked closer to the throne, I saw him as I had when we finally broke up that fall day so long ago. I saw him as needy. Needing me. The me I couldn't be for him. It made my love for Henry clearer, even in his absence. Even in my illicit daydreams, the truth was, I loved Henry.

"Honey, Julie always has been one of my biggest fans. She and I were almost in-laws. We have a bond. So, if you aren't available—which you've made it quite clear you aren't—what's the harm in Julie and me having a little fun?" Alex asked. His eyes glinted at me. "Scone?"

I rolled my eyes. This was my fault. I created this by letting him back in. "Alex, you're right. Have fun with Julie. I'm dying anyway," I said.

Both of us were silent, then, until—

"Whoa, passive-aggressive alert," Ralph said, barreling into my room as much as a man with stage four cancer and a walker could barrel. "I thought we talked about positive mental attitude and loving our spouses."

And then he stopped. Death-staring at Alex, Ralph said, "Hello, I'm Ralph Waldo Erikson, and you are?"

Alex seemed confused, as if I had a man ready to drop in at the slightest hint of conflict. Maybe I did. Maybe it didn't matter. Maybe nothing mattered. Alex extended his hand. "Alex Caldwell Thomas, if we're being that formal. Nice to meet you."

"Oh, you're the long-lost boyfriend, the early years, according to Jenn," Ralph said, settling into a brown chair. "This is good. See, it's hard for us to not glamorize the past, to not think of all of you, our past relationships, as perfect and to not criticize our current ones, no matter how good. We didn't get cancer with you, did we?"

"Ralph, please," I said. I didn't want this, didn't want truth or Alex—I just wanted to sleep.

Alex squeezed the paper Whole Foods bag in his hand and shot me an angry look. "Listen, Ralph. I didn't come here to challenge your knowledge of death or your knowledge of my old girlfriend. I just came here with bagels and cream cheese. To lighten the mood, so to speak," Alex said. "Want one?"

And to that, Ralph said, "Sure."

Of course, Ralph and Alex hit it off, talking art and history and travel—all of the topics I wished Henry and I spent time talking about, topics I wished Henry cared about. My eyelids kept growing heavy and by turn, Ralph or Alex would grab my hand in between stories, ostensibly to keep me awake. And maybe it was simply to keep me awake. It didn't work, though.

When I awoke again, Alex was sitting in a brown chair reading the paper, and it was late morning, at least that's what the news on the TV told me. I realized Ralph was gone. I'd need to apologize to him for my grumpy behavior and, of course, to find out what he thought about Alex.

"Good morning again, sleepyhead," Alex said, folding the paper and walking over to the throne.

"Tell me what's going on with Julie." I no longer had time to dance around subjects.

Alex sat down on the throne and smiled. "You and your sister are such special ladies," he said.

"What's that supposed to mean?" I asked.

"Just that, honey," Alex said. "You're the love of my life, and she's the next best thing to being with you."

"So you two are a couple? Have you slept together, you and Julie?" I asked, suddenly sure of it.

"Don't be silly, Jenn," Alex answered, looking at me as if I were a small child. "I've got to run, but I'm still planning on being back a little later to keep you company. It's our special weekend, and I wouldn't miss it for the world."

And with that, he kissed me on the lips and was gone, his folded newspaper a reminder of his presence.

Stripes brought in lunch and, surprisingly, it tasted like food. As I was eating, my wedding ring reflected rainbows onto the wall. Seven years ago, when Henry gave it to me, I was well, and everything was different. I had had no idea he would propose. We had just both needed a break, so we took a trip to California.

I had been without Alex for about a year, and Henry and I had become inseparable. In fact, at the time of the trip, I still couldn't believe the depth of our passion. My love-at-first-sight had lasted.

Neither of us had been to Big Sur before. We were astounded by the natural beauty, giddy with the thought that we had five days together. It was our first big trip as a couple, and we'd been talking about it and making plans incessantly.

The first night we'd arrived too late to make it to the beach for sunset, so we prepared by starting out early the second day. Driving through the small towns, towering trees, and sheer cliffs along Highway 1, we listened to Sting and Bono and laughed and talked. By three, we found a small deli, and Henry went inside to get food and wine while I sat in the rental car pinching myself.

"The most beautiful beach in the world is just down that road, according to Clyde in there," Henry said once he had put all of his purchases in the trunk.

"Perfect," I answered.

And it was. We spread a blanket on the sand, and I promptly fell asleep. When I woke up, the sun was drooping in the sky, peeking through the rock formations. Henry was sitting on the blanket next to me, grinning down at me.

"Did you sleep at all?" I asked, rolling onto my side.

"Nope, I couldn't," he answered. "I had something on my mind."

"You always have that on your mind," I teased but noticed he looked serious.

"Will you marry me?" he asked, pulling a gorgeous emerald-cut diamond ring out of his pocket.

I had never felt happier in my whole life as I said yes and he slipped the ring on my finger.

An hour later, Paige came in, pushing Hannah in the stroller and followed by Hank. She parked Hannah and Hank on the floor next to my bed and pulled a tub of wooden blocks from underneath the stroller.

Hank proceeded to build an impressive tower on the floor next to me. "It's your castle, Mommy," Hank told me. He looked happy. Hannah did too—she smiled up at me.

I was happy too, surrounded by life in its purest, most carefree form. Sometimes when Hannah looked at me with her baby-blue eyes, she seemed to understand the whole world; maybe she was still so close to God because she had only been on earth a little more than a year herself. For Hank, the fact that his mommy would go to heaven and be with God was somehow OK. God was good. Heaven was happy. I knew he didn't really understand, and his quiet acceptance broke my heart.

"How's it going in here?" Paige asked. She wore ripped jeans, a T-shirt with a peace sign, and huge diamond studs in her ears. She was a gorgeous, blond dichotomy—casual and fancy—in motion. She picked up Hannah. "Do you want her?"

"Sure," I answered. Paige had been great. It was so easy to take somebody for granted in this life, especially if that person was always there for you. Like Paige. I remembered how she and Jacob had worked forever to find me cute wigs when my hair fell out. On her own time, after she finished at my house, she was all over town. And makeup, she helped with all of that. Helped me feel and look better while being a blessing to my kids.

"Paige, I don't know what I would've done without you," I said as she plopped Hannah on the throne. Hannah wasn't in the mood to be snuggled, as usual, and pushed away.

"She's everywhere," Paige said, retrieving Hannah and standing her on the floor. Hannah clutched the bed for support and did a sideways shuffle toward Hank and his block castle, so universally appealing to babies.

"No, no, baby. No," Hank said, watching as the menace headed in his direction.

"Don't worry, Hank. She can't get to you yet," Paige said. "Hannah, let's go take a walk, OK?" And with that, Paige grabbed Hannah's two chubby hands and walked her out the door. "We'll be back in a few minutes, Hank."

"Bye!" he yelled cheerfully. He loved being alone with me almost as much as I loved having him to myself. "Mommy, when Daddy be back?"

The question, in its innocence, still hurt my feelings. Had Henry replaced me in Hank's heart? Is this how Juliana felt all those years when I asked for my daddy over her? "Soon, honey. Did you know we're having a big party soon?" I answered.

"Yes, a party for Mommy. To make you feel better."

�֍

After the kids left, I brushed my teeth and changed into a bright green sweat suit. I felt like visiting Ralph. Thoughts of our rainy-day sex Scrabble were dancing in my mind as I made my way down the hall. I thought I would ask Ralph about Alex, make sure he was on my side, make sure it was all right to see him again—if he even showed up again.

The only thing was, something inside told me telling Ralph anything about my feelings for Alex would be cheating not just on Henry but on Ralph as well. *What a mess.* I needed a man's perspective. But maybe, just maybe, now that Alex and Ralph had met, Ralph would have insights or guidance. Maybe?

I reached Ralph's door and stopped. His door was closed, which only happened when he was sick—really sick. How could that be? I'd just seen him. What was going on? Panic and dread rose in my throat as I tapped the door lightly, hoping to make it swing open. Success. The door creaked a bit, then obliged, exposing a pale and diminished Ralph and a startled Nurse Samuels by his bedside.

"Mrs. Benson," said Nurse Samuels with alarm. "Mr. Erickson isn't, um, doing very well. The family's been called. You may not want to visit right now."

Oh my god, I thought, moving as if underwater now. *This is it. The family's been called? Oh, Ralph.*

My ears were ringing as I approached his bed, ignoring Nurse Samuels. "I think he needs a friend right now. Is he in pain?"

"No, Mrs. Benson, the doctor just upped his medication."

I stood there, frozen beside his bed. Nurse Samuels moved behind me and supported me under my arm; I guessed she could tell my legs were about to give out.

I wanted to run from the sight and smell before me. The stale, mushed-bean smell. The drawn, jaundiced man on the pillow, lips parched and cracked at the corners. Where was Ralph? My vibrant, loving friend? The happy, successful businessman. Wonderful husband and family man. I searched for him in the curled-up form before me, head barely visible above the covers.

I found my voice. "Ralph, I'm sorry you aren't feeling well. You'll get over this. I love you, buddy…Please, get better, for both of us. I know…" My throat tightened and I couldn't go on. I couldn't stand the thought of not sharing my experience with Ralph. I reached for his thin, lifeless hand underneath the blanket and held it. It was so cold. Why was death so cold? Nurse Samuels pulled a chair over to me, and I gratefully sank into it. Then she left us alone.

"Please, Ralph, don't leave me," I cried, but it seemed too late. He had aged ten years in the few hours since I had seen him. Ralph squeezed my hand. A small little squeeze but a squeeze nonetheless. He knew I was there. He wanted me to let go. I wouldn't.

A noise at the doorway caused me to look up. Barbara and the kids were clustered in the doorway. For a moment, they looked afraid to come in. Then Barbara rushed over to the bed, followed by her two sons and daughter.

Barbara looked at me while her children absorbed the shock of their father's appearance, of what could be his final hours.

"Thank you," she said, and she leaned over and gently brushed Ralph's hair back from his forehead. Dismissing me, she was taking back her husband, taking charge of his last moments on earth. She reached for his hand. Fine, she could be the one to lose the tug-of-war with death, because I couldn't. I gave Ralph a final, determined squeeze and placed his hand firmly in Barbara's.

"Don't let go, Barb. Please," I said, struggling to stand, to make my feet carry me to his door. I heard his children breaking down into sobs as I left the room. I didn't look back.

9

Warning: Use professional driver in difficult conditions.
Avoid sharp turns and abrupt maneuvers.

I'D BECOME ADDICTED TO THE IDEA OF REMEMBERING, JUST LIKE
Henry was addicted to the game of golf. Of course, he wouldn't
understand. Wouldn't see the connection. Tough. He'd always told
me I needed a hobby, something to focus on outside work and the
kids. Now, I had two. Curing myself and remembering. Reliving
my past to stay alive. It was a full-time job, really, now. I got cancer.
It got me. But it doesn't define me, not yet. I had bad genetic luck,
but I'm a good person. Really, I am. I can remember, relive, the past
without being drawn back to it.

Everyone else got to be selfish. Take a break. I needed a break
too. Time away from being sick. Time away from being me now.

I wanted to be me then.

Me in college. With Alex. Carefree. Cancer-free.

Now was ruined anyway. Henry didn't really care about me anymore, did he? I mean, not like a wife, the person who would share
the rest of his life. Because he knew I couldn't be. I wouldn't be. I'd be
dead, and he'd be, well, alive, with our kids, and my daddy's business.

Before the cancer, we'd been growing as a couple and independently. Him with his practice. Me with my business. And then Hank. I do really believe kids can bring couples together or push them apart. Hank made us even more loving, more caring, more together. Until the cancer. His little hands in each of ours, completing our family circle.

I had loved having Hank in bed with us. Henry didn't, not so much. I could easily sleep through the little guy's sleep-time gymnastics—foot in the head here, a kick to the belly there—while Henry, the light sleeper, couldn't.

"Jenn, really, it's time for him to sleep in his crib," Henry said, poking me in the shoulder in the middle of the night. Little Hank, seven months old, was asleep on his back next to me, his head under my arm, his feet aimed at Henry's head.

"He's adorable—just look at him," I whispered about the sleeping cherub visible in the moonlight streaming in the window.

"He has a strong kick, and I have an early day tomorrow. I just want to sleep in my own bed, without getting kicked in the head. Please," Henry said. His eyes were ringed with dark circles from lack of sleep, and I felt sorry for him.

"OK, tonight, I guess," I answered. Henry moved quickly, picking up Hank in one swift motion, cradling him gently in his big arm. I watched as Henry tip-toed out of our bedroom and across the hall to Hank's nursery. It was so cute, seeing the big man with the tiny one.

"Finally," Henry said, coming back to bed after closing the nursery door and our bedroom door. He was asleep in an instant. I reached over and flipped on the baby monitor, missing the smell of Hank next to me in bed but enjoying the sleep sounds floating through the monitor. *Hopefully Henry will get a good night's sleep, and I'll have Hank back in our bed tomorrow night,* I thought before drifting off myself.

We laughed about the bed-hopping baby the next morning over coffee, but still we disagreed.

"I don't think you can ever get enough cuddle time," I said, reaching for Henry.

"Well, you've got me there," he said, before giving me a kiss.

We had shared so much, Henry and I. But now *we* didn't have anything. I had cancer. He had the kids, the house, the job, the golf, my daddy, my life before.

Now I had the ever-over-the-horizon hope for the cure, or the treatment that "prolongs life." I just had me, and being alone. Or, me, the burden of an otherwise blessed life. I was Henry's burden. His tithe for success, for our successes. This was our due, the reason we weren't connected anymore. He needed to be free of me, to be free.

My job was to disappear. To evaporate into the valley. Lying on my throne, becoming depersonalized. A pin cushion. A test pattern.

"Hello? Can I come in? Are you awake, Jennifer?" Alex said.

Oh my god, it's Alex. He's back. I needed him back.

Yes, I was awake. Drowning in self-pity, but nonetheless awake. "Alex?" I asked in a pathetic little voice.

"I'm sorry, Jennifer. I seem to be either too early or too late," Alex was saying. "I should've called first, but I just felt like I needed to hurry back, that you needed me. I'm not sure why. By the way, loved meeting your friend, Ralph, this morning. Great guy. Um, should I come back later?"

"No. It's fine. It's Ralph," I said. I couldn't keep those damn tears back anymore. I didn't mean for it to happen. Didn't mean to cry like a baby. "Sorry. It's just that Ralph may be dying, right now, down the hall. He's my best friend. Oh my god, his family is here. The doctors are here. They're trying to keep him alive. But I don't know if they'll win over death. And if he dies, I'll die, I just know it."

Alex grabbed me tightly around the shoulders. "Shhh, don't. Ralph will be fine, and you, you are not going to die, not now. You have so much more to do," Alex said. He wrapped his arms around me while I cried all over him, nose running, the whole works, until I could finally catch my breath. I clung to his now wet shirtfront and hoped it wasn't one of his favorites—soft and thick.

"What can I do? What would make these tears stop?"

"There's nothing." I shook my head. Where to begin? "I need to get out of here. I can't be here when Ralph dies. I can't. He can't die. I can't be here if he does. He is my only hope." And then I cried as if I hadn't ever cried. My body shook, and I couldn't stop.

Alex tried to hold me, but my shudders were too strong for him to hold. If he hadn't been there, I would've full-on wailed.

"How about this. I'll go check on Ralph's condition. I think one of those nurses is nice, right?" he asked, and because I couldn't answer, he disappeared out the door.

Ralph cannot die, Ralph cannot die, I told myself. *Please, God, please don't take Ralph. He is what I hold on to. He makes me strong. Without him, I am gone.*

I sat sobbing, waiting for Alex to return, and when he finally did, he was smiling.

"Honey, they think Ralph's going to pull through," Alex said. "I talked to some doctor, and he said Ralph would be fine. Maybe not right away, but eventually. Isn't that great news?"

I nodded, not trusting my voice, not quite believing Ralph could get better. I'd seen him, seen what he looked like, what death looked like.

"What would you think about getting out of here for a bit? Are you allowed?" Alex asked, sitting next to me, trying to look into my face. Lifting my eyes, I saw Alex's worried face, and I just wanted Ralph to be OK. I wanted to be gone from here. I wanted a break from this despair, from my life.

"Yes," I answered, sniffing. "I can leave, now. I want to leave here now. As long as Ralph is getting the attention he needs. They wouldn't let me in, wouldn't let me stay."

"There, there. When we get back, I'll force them to let you in to see him. Do I need to contact anybody? Sign you out or whatever?"

"I'll take care of it," I said, trying to quiet the gulping sounds I made whenever I had a really big cry. "But you have to realize, I'm not easy to take anywhere. I need to bring a lot of stuff, like that," I said, embarrassed to be pointing to my walker, sobs wracking my body.

"No problem. You just tell me what to grab, besides you, of course, and I'll get it. By the way, let's consider this a private party. I got your invitation, Jenn. There's no way I could ever go to a farewell party for you," Alex said. "So let's just get out of here for a while. Make it a better day, OK?"

"OK."

"Was that a smile?" Alex asked. "I'll pack whatever you need for the day. I'll get another Ralph update and be right back."

A few minutes later, Alex returned and told me Ralph had stabilized. He was no longer considered critical. The smile on Alex's face suddenly leapt onto mine. Ralph would be OK.

Alex said, "Get moving, Jenn. Our adventure awaits."

I was going somewhere, anywhere. Leaving Shady Valley for a day. I didn't even care where. Shower. Change. Pack. I'd leave a note for Ralph, so I didn't disturb him or make him worse when he wandered down to see me. I didn't want anyone worried. Ralph would understand why I had to go, and I'd be back before he knew it. He'd understand, he would. Wouldn't he? I hoped. It would be easier not to tell Henry, I reasoned. Let him golf. I'd be back long before he noticed I'd gone.

"Since when do you drive a Suburban?" I asked as Alex pushed the wheelchair up to the huge black truck.

"Since I have to haul you and all your equipment around, that's when," Alex said as he bent down, picked me up—effortlessly for such a slim, seemingly nonathletic guy—and deposited me in the passenger seat. "OK?"

"Great. It's great to be out here, outside. Thanks. By the way, where are we going?" I asked. Alex grinned and shut the car door without answering my question. I didn't care. I felt free. Almost giddy, really. I was wearing my pale-yellow sweat suit, to match Alex's sweater. Putting my Nikes on felt funny after months of just socks. It felt good to look dressed and normal.

I should've left more often, insisted that Henry take me home for a visit. He had offered, but I said it would be too sad to visit and not stay. He should have pushed me to leave Shady Valley, just like Alex did. Why didn't he? *Probably preparing our house for his new wife, new life,* I thought.

Alex was treating me like I was normal. Like it was normal for the two of us to be heading on an adventure together. On a summer Sunday.

"Ready?" he asked, hopping into the driver's seat. "Do you think we have everything?"

"I know, it's kind of hard for me to travel light," I said, embarrassed. I had to bring all of my medicine, my walker, my wheelchair, my special pillow, and so on.

"No problem, Jennifer. Really," Alex said, putting his right hand on my knee, pulling it away to put the truck in gear. "Sit back and enjoy the ride. We'll be there in a little while."

I looked out the window and saw Shady Valley as visitors must see it: a two-story, brick building in a bucolic setting of rolling hills. Mature evergreen trees surrounded the building and lined the drive, interspersed by perfectly manicured grass. The only giveaway that it was more than an oversized country schoolhouse was the illuminated emergency entrance sign pointing to the side of the building. Otherwise, something wonderful could take place inside those walls.

As we drove down the winding drive, fallen leaves swirled in front of us, a sign that fall was just around the corner. The hillsides were light-green and brown, scorched by the summer sun. I smiled, warm and happy, excited that Shady Valley was in the rearview mirror.

A wave of panic hit. *What am I doing leaving, with Alex, of all people? I should have called Henry to let him know,* I thought. *No, wait, that would've been stupid.*

I could have called Betsy, but she would have told me not to go. I wanted to go. I wanted to be here, with Alex, leaving Shady Valley, having an adventure. It would be fine. Everything would be fine. We were old friends, special friends who'd spent so much time together. If I wanted to spend quality time with Alex, well then, I would. I was.

I looked to my left and noticed Alex's smile. He saw me watching him and smiled more broadly. "What is it?" he asked.

"Oh, nothing, just thinking," I answered.

"About us?"

"About this. Is this a good idea?" I asked.

"It's the best idea," Alex answered, grabbing my hand and kissing the top of it. "And don't worry, my parents won't show up this time."

My stomach knotted, and I pulled my hand away. "Just friends, OK?" I asked.

"Of course," Alex answered, and clicked on the radio.

Somehow, I fell asleep on the drive, curled up in the front seat, my head resting on Alex's right leg. I awoke to the sound of crunching rocks under the tires of the truck. I should've known where we would go. It was a perfect idea, and yet I didn't think of it until we turned onto the gravel road.

"Good morning again, sleepyhead," Alex said, slowing to wave to the Fergusons, the caretakers who had watched over the Thomases' lake home as long as I'd known Alex. Alex waved again and yelled,

"Hi, you two," as he hopped out to open the gate. He hustled, I noticed. Probably didn't want them to know it was me in the truck. They had thought we'd get married too, I remembered.

The first time Alex invited me to his family's lake house, it had been a big deal. For me. It was the beginning of junior year in high school, and although I'd spent time with his parents before—they'd invited me to dinner at their home a few months after we officially started dating—I hadn't spent time with them under the same roof for an entire weekend. As I stressed about what to wear, what to pack, Alex kept reassuring me and trying to sneak a kiss as I moved around my room.

"Jenn, they love you already," he said. He was sitting on my bed, on my bright-pink comforter, watching me pack. Daddy would have killed him if he knew I had let him up in my room. He patted the empty spot next to him. "Come here."

"Alex, no, I need you to help me pack, so stop messing around," I said, feeling anxious. He winked at me. I'd never had a boy in my room before, and things were getting too intense. "Look, I'll just finish up. Can you come back in half an hour, and we can go?"

"Whatever," he said, his eyes betraying a flash of anger that his nonchalant comment tried to hide.

"I'm sorry," I mumbled, but he was already gone.

By the time he picked me up an hour later, he seemed fine. "I cannot wait to take you fishing, and cliff jumping, and hiking," he said as soon as I hopped in the car. "And guess what the best surprise of all is?" he added. "My parents aren't coming down until tomorrow, so we have the whole place to ourselves tonight. I told you not to worry about what to wear."

"But my mother thinks they're going to be there," I said, sounding like a baby.

"Don't worry. They'll never find out," Alex said, and something inside told me he'd planned this all along. I wasn't so sure. Our parents ran in the same social circles. Mine would kill me if they knew we were going to be alone.

The longer we drove, the more relaxed I became. Everything would be fine. My parents wouldn't have a reason to suspect anything, and Alex's parents would arrive in the morning.

We did go fishing and cliff jumping. I met the Fergusons, the caretakers, who seemed at ease with the notion that Alex's parents would be there "later."

That night, after I was settled into the guest room, after I had changed into jeans and a sweatshirt as the fall evening air cooled down, and as we were drinking a glass of champagne in the living room on an oversized brown leather couch, Alex suggested a dip in the hot tub. It had been a perfect day, a perfect evening, and although I knew he'd like more, we'd made a deal to wait.

"I'd rather just stay inside—this is wonderful," I said.

"The hot tub is warm, and you won't need any of this," Alex said, trying to tug my sweatshirt over my head. We wrestled on the couch, laughing, and somehow he managed to get the sweatshirt off.

Just as he leaned over to kiss me, the door swung open. His parents stood in the doorway. Thankfully, all we'd taken off was my sweatshirt. Although we looked guilty, I tried to tell myself we'd had a perfectly innocent day. Alex rolled his eyes before jumping up to greet them, giving me time to get myself together.

Now, considering the way the Fergusons were watching Alex, I realized they probably didn't know about Alex's quickie divorce. "Does she think I'm Cathy?" I asked as he hopped back into the truck.

"I'm not sure, but I just think it'll be easier if she doesn't know it's you, unless you'd like to say hi," he said.

"No, it's fine. I don't want to confuse them," I answered. *There are enough confused people here,* I thought.

The narrow gravel road was only wide enough for one car at a time and was just as I remembered it from so long ago. Steep, winding down the hillside until it opened up to a round circle driveway and the unassuming entrance to the lake house.

The house hugged the hill, saving its best features for lakeside. From the driveway, it seemed a rustic, cozy cottage; its weathered cedar shingles had long since aged to the gray of East Coast shore cottages.

When Alex opened my door, he said, "You're not surprised at all, are you?"

"Nope, I'm not. But I'm so glad you thought of this—to bring me here. We have so many memories here, at this house," I said, leaning forward and wrapping my arms around his neck. Aside from my blond head and his dark-brown one, we melted together like butter as he carried me to the door. How did he manage to unlock the door and hold me at the same time?

"Welcome home," Alex said, carrying me down the wide wood steps to the Mexican-tile great room, floor-to-ceiling windows glistening in front of us. Amazingly, leaves had begun to turn on some of the trees. Bright red. Soft yellow. I hadn't even noticed the colors, not from inside Shady Valley. Even the trees there were in a suspended state—evergreen.

"I don't remember it being so beautiful here, Alex," I told him as he plopped me down on the couch facing the windows. The chunky wood coffee table was the same—and the fireplace, with the stone mantel, suddenly brought back a flood of memories. "We had a lot of fun here, didn't we?"

"Especially times when Mom and Dad couldn't make it. Remember that long summer weekend? Your friends and their dates. My buds and theirs."

"Yes, and wine, and music, and shooting pool. Hey, where's the pool table?" I said, turning to look beyond the two-sided fireplace to where the pool table had been.

"With all of us grown and not using the house so much, Mom

turned that room into her writing and reading room," Alex said. "Sit tight—I'm going to unload everything."

All through school and until we broke up, every weekend, unless there was a football game or some other great party, we would come here with Alex's parents. I'd sleep in the guest bedroom, just up the first set of stairs, in a twin bed with a thick down comforter. Alex and his brother, his brother's friends, and his sister slept upstairs in the kids' wing. His parents' rooms filled the other half of the upstairs. Outside the windows, a wooden deck wrapped around the entire first floor and led down to a dock. Everything was comfortable. Lived in. Elegant.

The calm lake water was dotted with pollen and still, reflecting the colors of the leaves. Dragonflies. And stillness. A private lake in a private setting in a pristine part of the heart of the United States. The perfect place for me now. Shady valleys and glass-topped lakes.

I did it again. I fell asleep.

"Alex?" I called, waking to notice a lamp on in the corner of the room and darkness outside the huge windows.

"Good evening, sleepyhead. At this rate, we will have spent an entire day together and not even talked. Not that I mind it, of course. I always did like to watch you sleep," Alex said, walking over to my couch. I tried to sit up.

"I can't believe I missed the sunset," I said, wistfully. "What time is it?"

"You can watch it tomorrow night, if you'd like to stay that long," Alex said. "I bet you're hungry. Dinner's almost ready. I was thinking red wine—a nice burgundy, actually—to complement dinner. Sound good?"

"Sure," I answered, suddenly needing desperately to go to the bathroom and brush my teeth. "I may need help getting to the powder room. And yes, I'd love some burgundy."

"Are you feeling all right?" he asked, helping me to my feet.

"I feel right at home—so much so I can't seem to stay awake. I'm sorry. I guess the change of scenery is taking its toll," I said. He'd changed into a denim shirt and thick gray sweatpants. As I wrapped my arms around his waist, I smelled an indefinable cologne and the unforgettable aroma of Purina fish chow.

"You went fishing without me?" I said, suddenly even more upset I'd missed out on our day together.

"Just off the dock. I needed to stay close, in case you woke up. I didn't catch anything. I needed you to bring me luck," he said. "Why don't I just carry you, OK?"

Instead of taking me to my bathroom—the guest bath—Alex carried me up the second flight of stairs, up to the master bedroom suite, and gently parked me on the bed. From there, it was a short walk to the bathroom around the corner. The comforter was the same. Everything was the same, it seemed. Everything inanimate that is. We, of course, were both very much different. I had finally noticed his dark hair had flecks of gray, a dusting of time.

"I unpacked your stuff, and it's on the counter over there. I think you know where everything else is," he said, and for the first time, he blushed. It had been a long time since we'd been in this room together. The fan suspended from the two-story ceiling over the bed turned languidly, unimpressed with our sudden awkwardness. Why had he carried all of my things to this bedroom? Were his things in here too?

"Call me if you need anything," he said, pulling the door closed behind him.

My heart jumped. Alex's suitcase was on the floor on the other side of the bed. I reached for my walker. My heart pounded as I tried to shuffle across the thick off-white Berber carpet. I had a sudden new appreciation for those silly floors at Shady Valley. As I began to brush my teeth, I wondered what I was doing there, in the woods, in my old boyfriend's family's house. Me. A married mother of two. A happily married, dying mother of two.

I had to be going crazy. Temporarily insane. A side effect of the latest drug, perhaps? Extreme loneliness coupled with nostalgia and, I had to admit, desire. I loved Henry and our life, but something about Alex made me feel wanted in a way that I hadn't felt in a long, long time. I loved the way Alex made me feel like a woman again, instead of a sick person. But was it worth risking my marriage?

When he knocked on the door, I said, "Come in."

"A glass of wine for the lady?" Alex asked, crossing the room and placing the crystal flute on the marble countertop by the sink. "Do you need anything? Can I help?"

"No. Well, yes. Alex, why am I here? Why are we here?" I asked.

"I told you, we're having a party. I'm not coming to your other one, so this is it, kiddo. And I've missed you. You were my best friend for years. We need to catch up. Talk. Besides, you needed a break from that place, and poor Ralph."

"Yes. It's just that this room, this house. It all holds so many memories," I said. "I think I should be in the guest bedroom."

"No, this room is perfect. It's filled with good memories. Great memories, actually. Like the amazing-time time. Over there," Alex said, nodding toward the bed.

"Not like the first time in that horrible motel room," I answered, blushing.

"Look. It's not like you don't look cute in that canary yellow, but I think it's time for a change of clothes," Alex said, pulling a sky-blue cashmere pullover out of one of his mother's drawers. "And these," he added, holding up gray sweatpants much like his own. "May I?"

"There's really no need," I said, feeling self-conscious. I didn't want him to see all of my bruises. My surgery scars. My track marks.

"There's really no reason not to," Alex said, pulling up my sweatshirt before I had a chance to stop him. He pulled the soft sweater down immediately, saving me any embarrassment since he moved so fast. "Now then, my dear, let's drop your drawers." The entire process lasted a minute. And he was right: there wasn't any reason not to let him help me. We had been together countless times over the years. It was natural. Just friends. I squelched the rising panic in my throat. Where was this leading? And, the equally strong thought: I should go home.

"Brush your hair, put on a little makeup while I check on the steaks. I'll be right back," he said, dashing out of the room.

By the time he returned, my hair was smooth and shiny. My face, with a layer of powder, was matte. For a minute, looking at myself in Mrs. Thomas's mirror, I thought I could see a glimpse of the old me. The carefree me. Just a glimpse.

"You know, you're still just as beautiful as you were the day I felt my crush on you. The day I kissed you by the bicycle stand. At lunch. Remember?" Alex said, before picking me up again. Now it was my turn to blush.

"I remember," I mumbled. "Don't forget the wine."

"Never forget the wine," he said. "I hope you're hungry because I've made you a feast. Filet mignon, homemade mashed potatoes, and asparagus with hollandaise sauce. I hope it's OK if we eat out on the deck. It's a beautiful night, and I think fresh air will be good for you. That's what they always say, don't they?"

As he carried me into the long narrow kitchen open to the great room, all the smells hit me at once. Real smells. Real food.

"I want to light the candles. Can you make it the rest of the way, or do you need a lift?" he asked. He'd placed my walker within reach.

"I'm fine. I'll see you out there," I answered, making my way through the kitchen, the mud room, and finally across the threshold and out onto the wood deck. No shuffling on real wood, of course, because of the splinter risk. Alex had moved the table close to the door. I only needed about five steps. Three tiny citronella candles in terra cotta pots graced the table while at least fifteen larger citronellas were sprinkled across the deck. Candlelight reflected on the surface of the smooth lake. Every couple of minutes a fish jumped below, begging for fish chow. *Not tonight, fellows. Sorry.*

"You know what I've always wondered, Jennifer?" Alex said as he placed my plate in front of me. I think my stomach actually growled. "Tell me what Henry has that I didn't have."

I had just taken my first bite, and I felt my throat tighten. I forced myself to chew the meat slowly, afraid I would choke. I knew I had to choose my words carefully. "Timing, I guess," I answered, taking extra care to cut a small piece for my next bite of filet. I smiled and said, "This is so good."

"Yes, it is. Lots of things are good—were good. What does timing mean?" Alex asked.

"He came along at the right time. You and I had broken up, for good, as far as I knew. Heck, you already had another girlfriend by the end of that night," I answered slowly, hoping for a smile. "I had met Henry the summer before. I just decided to call him."

"You called him? Pretty bold for you," Alex said, swirling the wine in the crystal glass. "You must've really wanted him."

10

Warning: Not to be taken internally. Avoid contact with face.

HIS TONE HAD AN ICY QUALITY I HADN'T HEARD BEFORE. I IG-nored it and launched into the familiar story of my first lunch date with Henry, as if we were old chums just catching up. I ignored his panther eyes flashing dangerously at me across the candlelit table.

"I called him with a legal question, he asked me to lunch, and I said yes. He asked me how you were doing, and I told him we'd broken up. Then I asked him how his long-distance love was, and he told me they were engaged. I wanted to jump out of the car," I said. I had been devastated. Here I was, boldly calling the first and only guy I'd ever pursued, and he was engaged to somebody else.

"But you didn't want to run back to me?" Alex asked, his mood darkening. I'd only seen him like this a few times before—and it wasn't good. Those eyes, that version of his eyes, were the reason we weren't together anymore, I finally realized.

"Sometimes I did. But you were dating Cathy by then. I had to move on too," I said.

"You could've chased me for once," he said. "But no, you decided to chase somebody else, a nobody redneck engaged to somebody else. That makes a lot of sense."

"Henry's not a redneck," I said quietly.

"Sure he is. But so are you, when you think about it. New money. Burgers." His steak knife was frozen in his right hand.

"What's wrong with you, Alex?" I asked. I had stopped eating, and to keep my hands from shaking had clasped them below the table.

"You ruined my life. You left me. And, the next thing you know, you're married. To a redneck. Having his babies. The life I always dreamed we'd have. I spent the best years of my life courting you. And then what'd I do? Married the first bimbo I dated after dating you. Moved to goddamn Texas, of all places," Alex said, his voice loud now, his mouth drawn taught—but he was very still, except for swirling the wine in his glass.

"Alex, you're making me nervous. I've always loved you. You're such an important part of my life, my whole life," I said, trying to calm him down. Turn him back into the Alex I'd always known. The mellow, trusting, and calm Alex. The Alex who was always there. Always reliable. And back into the Alex who always had adored me, pursued me, forgiven me.

"I knew it, Jennifer. I knew you felt the same way. My life is nothing without you. The happiest memories are all with you," he said. Then he added softly, "and my worst. More wine?"

"Sure," I said, thinking I better find a way to make it disappear, maybe through the cracks of the decks or in the potted plants. He'd definitely had enough. I hoped we were returning to safer ground. I watched his face in the flickering light as he continued.

"Do you know what Cathy said to me the night she left me for her rich cowboy? Do you know? She said I was boring. Too dependable. Too supportive. Too nice. And where'd it leave me? Alone in a cheesy suburb of Dallas, with no trees, no roots, no culture, and eventually, no wife. I'm just forgetting that part of my life," he said, making eye contact with me again. "That's what I've done. I want to go back to you and me. You can't deny you feel it too. You wouldn't be here if you didn't. If you're so damn happy, then why are you here with me, Jenn?"

"I'm sorry, it was obviously a mistake," I said. "After dinner, you can take me home. We'll have this great memory to share. I need to check on Ralph and well, you know."

"You always were sorry, weren't you? And you've always got something better to do with someone else. Remember when I surprised you junior year in college? Drove down to see you. All your roommates were so good about lying to me, you know, about the others, that I really believed you were still all mine. What an idiot. I should've known you couldn't be faithful. So I called you. Told you to meet me in ten minutes for dinner. And what did you do?"

He stood up, leaning forward over the table.

"For God's sake, Alex, that was in college, almost fifteen years ago! We've been over these same things a million times. Why do you think we couldn't make it? You can't let anything go!" I said, sliding my chair back from the table.

"You cheat on me for four years, and it's my problem?" he demanded. His eyes flashed, and his jaw muscle flexed. I couldn't believe we were having this fight again. We weren't dating anymore. He had no right to bring this up, no claims on me. But for the first time in my life, I felt physically threatened by a man, and I tried to keep my voice reasonable.

"I had a date," I stated. "I told you we should date other people. You agreed."

"No. I told you to do what you wanted. I'd do the same. And you know what I did?"

"No," I said, standing up. A stranger on a dark side street. That's what Alex was becoming before my eyes.

"I followed you around that weekend. I watched you on your date. Flirting with the loser guy. Hell, his pants didn't even fit, but I guess that was part of the appeal. And I followed you to the woods, where you went with him. How could you, Jennifer? Didn't our love mean more than that?" he said, still leaning forward, gulping the last of his wine. "I need some more wine. I'll be back."

What else had he done that I didn't know about? What else had he watched? I needed to get back to Shady Valley. This was all a big mistake. Suddenly, I knew I would be safer inside, away from the open flames and the black quiet water. Away from the edge. With uncharacteristic strength, I allowed the adrenaline from my pounding heart to propel me inside.

Alex and I met at the doorway. "Cold?" he asked.

"Yes. Could we talk inside?" I asked.

"Sure, Jennifer, whatever you'd like, as always," he answered.

"You better blow out the candles, just to be safe," I suggested.

"Yes, I'll do that. You just go on inside and make yourself comfortable," he said.

I felt foolish, but I needed to get to a room with a lock. And a telephone. As I hurried as much as I could through the kitchen, I realized the closest sanctuary would be my old room, the guest room, at the end of the long hall, across the great room from the kitchen. I could do it. *Halfway there—*

His hand grabbed my shoulder. "Jennifer, where are you going?"

"Oh, ah, just to the bathroom," I answered as he picked me up.

"Let's go on up. That'll be more fun," Alex said. He was humming to himself as he carried me up the stairs. "So, wondering what else I know about, Jennifer?"

"You're making me nervous. The veins in your neck are sticking out," I said. He swayed but caught himself by leaning on the wall.

"That's what you do to me. You drive me crazy. You always have. You're such a self-centered bitch, but I happened to love you. I did, Jennifer. We could've had such a wonderful life together. But you couldn't be faithful to me, and it seems, you can't be faithful to poor ol' Henry, either. Well, his loss is my gain, as they say."

He was looking into my face with enraged eyes, unrecognizable, swaying in the middle of his parents' bedroom. I couldn't speak. The ceiling fan creaked as it swirled far above us.

"Alex, please believe me," I pleaded. "I never wanted to hurt you. Please. Let's calm down."

Alex forced a strange, high-pitched laugh and tossed me roughly on the bed. Tears sprang to my eyes as I searched in vain for some object that might come to my aid on the night table. Then Alex was on top of me, pinning my head to the bed by my hair, holding my wrist too tight with his other hand, pressing his lips against mine. I couldn't breathe.

Just as suddenly, Alex pulled off of me. "Yeah, baby, I know how you like it." He growled, now pressing both wrists to the bed with his hands. "I could show you. I could."

Great gulping sobs wracked my body. Pain seared through me, and my head began to pound.

"Crying? You're crying? You're pathetic," he mumbled. Releasing me, his anger spent, he rolled over to lie panting beside me.

With trembling legs, I slid off the bed and stumbled into the bathroom, locking the door behind me. My tear-streaked face mocked my romantic fantasy of a "date" with my past love. How could I have been so stupid? So unfaithful to Henry?

I turned toward the big glass shower. If only I could wash away my sins. I turned the water on high and stepped into the soothing spray. The hot water streamed over my throbbing body while a thousand emotions raced through my mind. What if Alex wanted more? What if he was out there, waiting to kill me?

In a way, that might be easier than going back and facing Henry. What would I tell Henry?

11

Warning: If pain or fever persists, consult a physician because these could be signs of a serious condition.

EMERGING FROM THE SHOWER AT LAST, I WRAPPED MYSELF IN one of the Thomases' luxurious towels and reached for the wall to steady myself. The steam from the hot shower had left me light-headed, and for a moment I felt the room tilt. When I trusted myself to walk, I inched carefully forward, opened the door, and peered into the bedroom. Alex was gone.

I spotted my yellow sweat suit in a heap on the floor and quickly pulled it on, shivering. I prayed for someone to come to the house. The Fergusons up the road. Alex's parents. A rescue team sent by a worried Ralph. Henry.

Maybe not Henry. What would he do if he found me here, like this? Beat Alex up? Leave me?

I eyed the phone in the bedroom, but who could I call? What would I say? I came to a remote cottage with an ex-boyfriend, and he got the wrong idea—well, duh. I had no choice. I had to find Alex and convince him to take me back to Shady Valley. My stomach turned.

I saw him as soon as I started down the stairs. Out on the deck, staring out at the water. No way was I going out there again. The thought of that cold, black water and Alex's cold, black eyes made my heart race in terror. At the bottom landing, I stopped. "Alex." I tried to sound calm, normal.

He continued to stare at the water, and I thought he hadn't heard me. Suddenly, he grabbed a plant from the deck railing and threw it in the water.

I screamed before I could cover my mouth. As he reeled to face me, I could see the anguish in his eyes.

"Dammit, Jennifer, it wasn't supposed to be like this. You have to believe me. I didn't mean…I didn't want it to be this way. I didn't want to hurt you. You have to know that—you have to," he pleaded.

"If that's true, then please take me back, Alex, now. Tonight. I need to go back."

He nodded slowly and pushed away from the railing. "I guess you're right, Jennifer. We really aren't good for each other anymore. Maybe we never were. I'll go get your stuff."

I surveyed the great room for what I knew would be the last time. Some adventure. A trip to hell with the past as guide.

He was back. He bent to pick me up, but I bristled at his touch.

"No, thank you, Alex, I can manage." I said, and I did, though somewhat slowly. Once I reached the Suburban, however, I had to admit I needed help hoisting myself into the huge front seat. I scooted as far to the right as possible and clung to the door.

We drove back through the gates and along the winding road in silence that stretched for miles. Suddenly, I had to know. "How long have you been planning this?"

"Jennifer, I already told you. I didn't plan for it to get out of hand like that. I thought you wanted me too. You sent out some pretty strong signals back at your place, you know. I—something—just snapped. Being back in that house, thinking about the past, it was too much. You've got to forgive me, Jennifer. I can't go back to Cathy until I know you do," he said.

"What? I thought she left you? For another man," I stammered.

"No, not yet. We'll be divorced soon. I dropped everything to be here for you. Like always, when you needed me, I was there. You did need me, Jennifer. You just got a little more of me than you bargained for," he said. "Oh, and about Ralph. Nice guy, but I sort of lied. I couldn't get anyone to tell me his condition, and I knew you wouldn't leave unless he was stable. So I just told you he was. Consider it payback."

Oh my god. Ralph wasn't stable? I stared in disbelief, wondering if his remorse was as real as his story about Ralph or the oil baron. At least I knew, thankfully, this would be our final good-bye. If nothing else, then, I had closed one door at last. Did I actually feel sorry for him then? No, not at all. I felt nothing for him but darkness.

We rode the rest of the way in silence. What was there to say? He parked the Suburban in the loading zone and hopped out of the car. I sat frozen, still digesting his last words. He opened the door and helped me out. Then he unloaded all of my equipment and placed it on the curb next to me.

"Please forgive me and think about what I said. I don't want to leave you—us—like this."

"You got what you wanted, Alex. Now leave." I met his gaze defiantly, free to be angry at last.

"At least let me help you inside, Jennifer—it's the middle of the night."

"Just go, get out, goddammit, you've done enough, lied enough! I'll ring the nurses. Go back to Texas and your bimbo wife. Tell her all about your nice visit back home." I was shaking now, but I wasn't about to let him make me cry again.

He stood uncertainly for a moment but turned and headed back to the black Suburban. As he drove out of my life for good, I pressed the nurse call button by the door.

And that's when my legs gave out, and I crumpled onto my belongings. That's where Nurse Hadley found me. She sounded her pager alarm, and within a minute, the staff of Shady Valley was there, loading me onto a stretcher and mumbling among themselves, trying to understand if I had been coming or going.

They rolled me into the inpatient intensive care room, and the on-call doctor hurried into the room, and someone tried to change me into a gown, and Nurse Hadley said, "Look at her. She's got bruises on her wrists. I think she's been attacked."

12

Warning: May cause drowsiness.

No one asked me what happened. No one. Not Dr. Chris. Not the nurses, not Henry or Daddy, who arrived back here in the middle of the morning, a day early from Philadelphia. I slept through most of his visit, so Henry went home to take a shower, telling the nurses he'd be back. Mother called twice to check on me.

But nobody asked me what happened.

"You were attacked, Jennifer," Dr. Chris said. I nodded. Was that a question, or just a statement of fact? Did he think I was on a date? Did he blame me too? I supposed he should.

"The good news is you'll be fine, just a few bruises. If you take it easy, you should recover, physically, but I'd suggest you and Henry talk to a counselor. Quite often, deep emotional scars are left—on both the victim and the spouse of the victim," Dr. Chris added, making sure to stay busy checking my vital signs. Sure not to make eye contact. "I'd also suggest notifying the authorities. It doesn't seem possible you were abducted by a stranger, so you will need to identify your attacker. Get some rest."

"Chris, how is Ralph? I need to see him," I said.

"Oh, Jennifer," Dr. Chris said, suddenly finding something interesting in the corner of my ceiling. Then he turned to me and said the words I was dreading: "Ralph passed away last night. We tried everything, but it was his time. I'm so sorry—I know how close you were. I'll give you some privacy," he added, turning and leaving the room.

Nobody was talking about me or to me because Ralph died. Ralph. Died. I left Shady Valley on the day Ralph needed me the most. I abandoned my best friend. Oh my god.

There was a light knock on the door. It was a polite Pastor Barker knock. He didn't know. Or maybe he did. "Jennifer? Can I come in?"

"Of course, Pastor Barker," I said.

"Can I be of help?" he asked.

"I hope so, because if you can't, I don't know who can," I said between sobs. I needed to tell someone—someone had to know the truth. I told him what had happened. "I feel so guilty. I thought he was a friend, a true, lifelong friend. I was lonely, feeling sorry for myself. I never meant for anything like this to happen. What do I tell Henry? And I left Shady Valley on the day Ralph needed me the most, and now he's dead. It's all my fault."

"My goodness, you've found yourself a mountain of trouble," Pastor Barker said, sitting back in the brown chair, needing a moment to absorb his lost sheep's revelation. "Ralph did not die because of you. I was there, with him, with his family. He was at peace at the end. You wouldn't have been permitted into the room anyway. I suspect that's how you left here unnoticed, as we were all very focused on Mr. Erickson."

"The way I should've been," I cried.

Pastor Barker ignored me and continued, "I am sorry you've encountered this betrayal by your so-called friend. Such evil. Tell Henry what happened as you told me. Tell him that you weren't interested in romance, just friendship, when you agreed to spend the day with this man," Pastor Barker said. "Do not let what this monster has done come between you. I suggest you and Henry plan some time away together. After you get your strength back. It would do you both good. I think, maybe, that's what led you into this trap. You just need a break from fighting for your life. You need to feel God's grace and embrace."

"Why wasn't he there for me yesterday? I prayed. I begged for his help. I didn't think I asked for that much. I didn't even ask for a cure. All I wanted was to be free, to be back here, with Henry and the kids."

"Jennifer, you are here. God doesn't control everyone, but he does know about everything. He knows who can handle what. You became a victim of someone else's twisted reality. That wasn't God's work. God brought you safely back here, and God will grant you peace. He'll grant Henry peace as well. Shall we pray?"

"Yes, I guess we should," I answered.

I wondered if Pastor Barker got the chills when Julie crossed his path in the hallway. He wouldn't know she was my sister. She appeared moments after he left. Since then, I'd been trying to stay afloat. I read the only way to survive quicksand is to lie on your back and slowly do the backstroke to the edge of the pit. That's what I'd do now, during her visit: lie flat, hope she'd leave before I went under.

"I talked to Alex this morning," Julie said, unfolding Jacob's butterfly chair and pulling it over next to the throne.

I know I'm tired and bruised, but I think she just mentioned Alex—

"I should've told you he wasn't right, that he was a little depressed," she said, not making eye contact. "You really shouldn't have led him on, as usual, Jenn. I mean, really, haven't you tortured him enough? Alex and I were just starting to have so much fun—and, as usual, you ruin things."

"What are you saying?" I asked, wondering what she knew, what she and Alex had together.

"When Alex called me last week and told me he was in town for a visit, we went out for coffee together, to catch up on old times," Julie said, casually examining her manicured nails. "You know, I was always his sounding board, reassuring him when you strayed or whatever. I always liked him. Anyway, he seemed different somehow. Preoccupied. It was something in his eyes. I remember hoping he was drinking decaf. He seemed uptight. I should've warned you, but you seemed so happy he was back. Well, that, and he and I had so much fun together. At dinner, at the house, he really couldn't keep his hands off me. It was crazy."

I closed my eyes. I was the crazy one. How could she be here, telling me this now? Why did she wait until it came to this? A chill swept through me.

Julie kept talking. "The nurse told me they think he attacked you, took you away from here against your will. That's just not possible, is it, Jennifer? Alex wouldn't do that—I know he wouldn't, would he? Jennifer, I know you don't want Henry to know the truth, but you can level with me. Whatever happened, it happened because you wanted it to, for old times' sake, right? Secretly, you've always been a little slutty."

"Did Alex send you?" I asked, opening my eyes, staring at my sister. I moved my arms and legs a little to stay afloat.

"Of course not. He left town," she answered.

"I don't believe you, but here is the truth. I chose to go with him," I admitted. And maybe it was all my fault. I'd toyed with Alex too long, for too many years, and when he reappeared in my life, I was ready to use him again. He just used me better. *He loved me more then,* I thought. *He hates me more now.* No, that's not true—for once, the feeling was mutual. "You know, he's not even really divorced. At least, not yet. You really should watch what you're getting yourself into, especially when you're dealing with hand-me-downs."

Julie's eyes widened. "Well, I know what he's been going through, Jenn. And I know how much you put him through all those years.

Just try to understand how he must feel—I know he wouldn't hurt you on purpose. He's such a love."

"I need to rest. Can you leave, please?" I asked, trying to stay calm.

"Right. Sure, focus on your party, why don't you? Wendy Hinton called yesterday, from Cleveland, and she wants to come see you before the party. And Liza McBride, she's flying in from out west or somewhere. Anyway—"

"Julie, just get out!" I yelled.

Jacob blew in past Julie. "Oh my god, Jennifer. I called, and they wouldn't put me through, and I demanded to know what was going on, as your partner, and one of those nurses said you'd been attacked," Jacob said. After hugging me, he turned to Julie. "Surprised to see you here."

"Just leaving, actually," Julie said.

"I don't trust her, Jennifer," Jacob said. "Are you all right?"

"Jacob, I need to rest—can you check on Ralph? I need to see Ralph," I said, unable to keep my eyes open any longer. Mercifully, Dr. Chris had upped my meds to help me handle both the pain and the guilt, I think.

"OK, sure. I'll check on Ralph, sweetie. You just rest, OK? We had another record day Saturday, by the way. I love you, and I'll check on Ralph. Be right back," he added, kissing me on the top of the head.

"You need to eat, honey; otherwise, they'll tube you," Henry whispered into my ear.

How romantic. Tubing. Like the time I spent in Colorado, the summer in Boulder. With Lynne, another high school buddy, watching her aunt and uncle's house and farm while they went on an extended family trip. I still remember that cold mountain stream water, the sun surging through the breaks in the trees, the white warnings of the small-stream rapids. Making it to the bottom without tipping.

"Jennifer, wake up," Henry said, again pushing through my dreams like a diver cutting through calm water.

"Hi," I said, opening one eye. He looked calm. But I knew it was coming. The reaction. Would he pretend nothing happened, thereby blaming Alex? Or would he ask me why I would leave without telling him? Would he be jealous? Furious? Sad? Heartbroken? And what was I feeling? Abandoned? Lonely? Unloved?

"Did Ralph die?" I asked. "I had a bad dream that Ralph died."

"Honey," Henry said, reaching for my hand. "Yes, Ralph is gone."

There it was. Confirmation. My best friend. Gone.

"Paige said she's bringing the kids over tomorrow afternoon for Barney and a snack, if you're up to it. She'll call first," Henry said.

What if he really means, "Where do we go from here?" I guess he goes to work, makes more money, and finds that thin brunette attorney to call his own, I thought.

"So, how are you feeling? Can I bring you anything?" Henry asked, turning and walking across the room to the chairs. He grabbed the closest one and dragged it over beside the throne. Suddenly, I had a mental picture of Alex in the same position.

"I'm fine, really, Henry. I'll be fine. Well, who the hell knows? I'm dying of cancer, but otherwise, I'll be fine," I answered.

"That's why I just want you to get some rest. The kids need their mom feeling OK for their visit," Henry said, reaching out to hold my hand.

"Okeydokey, I'll be fine," I answered, turning to look at the closest green-striped wall. Henry was acting weird. Really weird. I couldn't take it anymore. His kindness. "Listen, here's the truth. I was lonely. I have been lonely, Henry." I knew I had to pick my words carefully, but I also needed Henry to understand how I felt. Why I left, even if I didn't understand everything myself. "Alex asked me if I wanted to go for a drive. I said yes."

"Why don't we talk about the 'drive' later. You've had a big loss, and from what Dr. Chris said, physical injuries to deal with," Henry said evenly.

"Henry, Pastor Barker suggested that we talk, talk now," I said, looking into his eyes, searching for him. His face was a mask.

"Well, the helpful Shady Valley crisis counselor told me I needed to help you deal with your loss, Ralph's death, since, as she put it, you're probably in shock," Henry said. He had started pacing at the foot of my bed. "Do you think you're in shock, Jenn? I think I'm in shock too. So maybe we shouldn't talk at all?"

"Henry, I'm so sorry, it was just a drive, a short excursion away from here," I said to his back.

"A drive? You packed a fucking suitcase, Jenn," Henry said, turning around and banging his fist on the throne. "You don't pack for a drive, do you?"

"Sit down, Henry," I said and noticed my hands were shaking. His anger was stirring up everything that had happened with Alex. I felt light-headed. "I will not be talked to like that. I will not be yelled at by you or anyone else. That's the last thing I need right now."

Henry sat down, and we were both silent. I remembered Pastor Barker's advice about telling the truth. *I owe it to Henry to try to explain,* I decided. It would be up to him to believe me—or not.

"Don't you get it?" I said quietly. "I've been lonely. You are at work or out of town, enjoying life, living, and I'm here, in this stupid place, so when an old friend asks if I want to go for a drive, then I say yes. That's what happened."

"That's not 'what happened,'" Henry said darkly, making quotation marks with his fingers. "What happened was that you left here with your old boyfriend for a romantic getaway the minute I left town. That's 'what happened.'" Tears welled up in his eyes, and he brushed them away.

I'd try again to make him understand, to make him believe me, the way I needed him to believe. "Alex drove me to his parents' lake house. I had no idea we were going there. I didn't pack a suitcase, but Alex did, in case I needed a change of clothes, that's all."

Henry looked into my eyes. "Bullshit, Jenn. That's bullshit."

I ignored Henry's outburst. "He made me feel like we were just old friends, catching up. That it would just be a dinner, and that's it. But then he attacked me and dumped me on the sidewalk outside," I said, my voice quivering a bit with the memory, tears stinging my eyes.

Henry looked down at his hands, clenched in his lap. I kept staring at the top of his head, praying he'd look up, look at me. See me.

"Henry, it's all over now. I just want to plan a trip for us. As soon as I feel stronger. I want to go to Napa Valley. Stomp grapes. Drink wine. Ralph said it's harvest time there, you know? We haven't been together, outside of here, in so long. That's all we need. We need to find each other again. Ralph is down the hall, fighting for his life. He can't even get out of bed. God, why won't anyone tell me how he is doing?"

"Jenn, Ralph—I—" Henry said.

"I'm still here," I said, interrupting. "I can still go somewhere, do something. We can still find each other again. Please."

Henry's hands were opening and tightening, opening and clenching. Finally, he looked up and into my eyes. "Jenn, Ralph is dead. I am so sorry about that. I know what he meant to you. I also know what Alex means to you, but I'm going to have to get the police involved. Where did he hurt you, Jenn? I can't just —"

"Can't what?" I asked. "You can feel hurt, even violated, betrayed, but it's my decision to call the police. My life's too short for all of that. Please," I said.

Finally, he grabbed my left hand with his. Henry's hands were big and rough, like bear paws. He was a white collar guy with blue collar hands. I thought of Alex calling him a redneck and felt angry for not standing up for him more. At least he knew how to work. Alex had been handed everything in his life, and look at him. Henry sat silent again, thinking. Reasoning, no doubt, that he could exact his revenge later. When I was gone. Secretly, I hoped he did. I'd brew up a big thunderstorm and take some pictures. In the meantime, I needed to go to the wine country.

"Did you know Ralph and Barb went out of town, and it really helped them work things out?" I asked, realizing that was the last trip Ralph would ever take. Henry knew they were fighting—he'd heard about it from me. What I was just realizing was that we should have been fighting too. Instead, we had both been pretending things were OK in our relationship. They weren't. Not after what I'd done with Alex. Not before.

Henry began pacing again, across the very spot in my room where I'd enjoyed a romantic picnic with Alex. My stomach turned at my betrayal. At my duplicity. At my need for attention at any cost.

I sat up and climbed slowly down from the throne. Even with the extra pain medication, I ached in every joint. Henry watched me but didn't come toward me to help. I made my way to where he was standing, watching me, from the center of my room, from the picnic place. "I am so sorry, Henry. I was wrong. I thought I was getting out of here, but I got myself in trouble. Nothing happened. I'm back now. All we need, you and I, is time alone, away from here. I just know it." I reached up and touched his face, and he finally looked down at me and brushed my hair behind my right ear.

"You're a pain in the ass, and I still don't understand why you left here with him," he said, hugging me. Finally. "But you're right. I'd like to get you away from here. We'll go to Napa when you are better," he said. "And don't leave here without me ever again. Promise?" He scooped me up then, carrying me back to the throne, gently placing me on top of the bed.

"Promise. Henry, shouldn't we talk about what happened?" I asked. I didn't want to ask, but if Pastor Barker was right, we really needed to talk it out, and I didn't think we had, not at all.

"We'll talk later," he said, rubbing his gold wedding band. The tie that binds. The bond Alex could never break. "I love you."

"Henry, can we talk about it now?" I repeated.

Henry looked at me then, and he had tears in his eyes again. "I'm sorry I wasn't here for you, babe," he said. "I should've been here, not golfing. I should've protected you."

"It's not your fault. I've taken you for granted. Ralph says I should be saying thank you and that I love you more. He's right. You've always been there—I'm sorry you had to cut your trip short," I murmured. *Wake up. Wake up.* "I am so sorry. This is all my fault. Not yours. All mine." *Why can't I keep my eyes open?*

"Before you go to sleep, sweetie, please tell me you didn't sleep with him," Henry said.

"No, no sleeping," I murmured.

"Get better," Henry whispered.

"Let's leave tomorrow," I said—or maybe I dreamed that.

13

Warning: Not suitable for all audiences.

THE NEXT MORNING, HENRY ARRIVED AND FOUND ME STARING AT the television. I could feel his anger in the way he silently and oh so politely went about tidying my room. *The strong but silent act,* I thought as I watched him. *Maybe he should just tape a scarlet* A *on me and get it over with.* All the silence and attempts to be civil had to be killing him on the inside, and I knew he was a time bomb just waiting to go off. I'd had enough of men and pent-up anger issues. I wasn't going to take this from Henry.

"OK, let's talk," I said. Henry's back was to me. He didn't say anything.

I focused on the TV screen. The anchor's lips were moving, but I wasn't really listening. Instead, I was imagining a different scenario. "This just in from Shady Valley in Columbus, Ohio. Ralph Waldo Erickson is dead after his brave fight against cancer. If you were too busy to come see him while he was still alive, don't miss the funeral and your last chance to feel better. We hear his best friend deserted him on the very day he needed her most. So sad, really. Again, local great guy Ralph Waldo Erickson is dead at age forty-five." I shook my head.

Ralph would be fine. I'd be fine. We would all be fine. *No, Ralph was dead,* I reminded myself. I just couldn't believe it—still.

"I told you, we can talk later. I just don't feel like getting into it right now," Henry said, finishing his tidying, settling into a chair, and opening his book.

"Well, maybe I do feel like talking about it," I said, crossing my arms, doing a perfect imitation of a toddler. "I hate this silent treatment."

"It's not really your choice this time, Jenn. It's mine. You are the one who left with your old boyfriend. I'm the one who has to deal with it," Henry answered, keeping his back turned toward me.

So much for talking, I thought. "Can you take me to see Ralph? No one will take me to his room. Nurse Hadley said I needed to rest. What I need is to see my best friend. Please, Henry?" Henry looked at me and shook his head.

I had a new theory that, if I escaped to California, even for a weekend, everything would be fine. The bad would be gone. No Alex. No cancer. Ralph believed in the power of California—for what good it did him.

And then there was the subject sitting between us like an overweight airline passenger who needed a belt extender. My duplicity. I had no idea if or when Henry would find it in his heart to forgive me, let alone talk to me about it. Maybe I'd find my miracle, and it would be forgiveness. I turned my head away from Henry and burrowed into my pillow so he couldn't see the tears. Across the room, sitting in my brown chair, Henry was absorbed in a book. Judging from its thickness, he could stay that way for days—a silent, judging, reading watchdog.

"Henry, I just think maybe a trip would—"

"Jenn," he interrupted. He closed the book, crossed the room, and pulled me toward him, hugging me for only the second time since he had returned from Philadelphia. Since Alex. He kissed me too—a passionate, deep kiss that stirred feelings deep inside me. *Wow.* A dating kiss.

"I love you, and you know how sorry I am about Ralph, and for leaving you alone. I know you were scared. You are scared. You aren't Ralph—you aren't going to die, not while I'm around."

"I love you so much. I'm so sorry," I said, still tingling from the unexpected passion.

As I held his hand, I turned again to look outside. Things would work out. The kiss reassured me and made the elephant between us seem to disappear. We settled into an easy silence then, watching the news together.

I thought about the days ahead. How much I should or could tell Henry. Could he handle the truth about what happened with Alex? Did I even know the truth? Maybe his way of handling it was better after all. I had screwed up my end of the marriage bargain, while he had more than upheld his. He got bonus points for the sickness part. How could I possibly tell him the truth without tearing us apart? I couldn't, I decided. No way. Talking might make me feel better and him worse, much worse. I read about that before somewhere. It was never smart to admit to an affair.

If I admitted to the attraction I had felt for Alex and the escape he offered, Henry would leave me. No more passionate kisses. No second chances. I needed Henry to see me as a woman, as his lover, and not just as his sick wife and a burden. But my need for him to feel that way about me didn't make it right to cheat on him with Alex. What had I done?

We didn't hug or kiss again, although I did try to initiate a hug. Henry pulled away and patted my hand. *Let the games begin*, I thought.

"Jenn," Henry said. I was relieved he was finally ready to talk. "I need you to understand, to accept that Ralph died. I'm worried that you aren't processing the fact of his death. Should I bring the counselor in here? I know you feel guilty because he died the night you were with Alex," Henry said, staring up at the ceiling as I turned to stare at him.

"No, no, he didn't," I answered. "He was fine when I left, rebounding. Alex told me he was stable. That's the only reason I left. I need to go see him. Why won't anyone let me go see him?"

"Jenn, he's gone. The funeral is in two days. We'll go together," Henry said. "I'm so sorry."

Ralph gone? Gone. Dead. *This is my fault,* I thought. I left him when he needed his best friend. I went to the stupid lake house with stupid Alex. I'm an idiot. "Nooo!" I wailed as Henry held me tight.

At some point, Nurse Hadley was in the room, and with a shot in the arm, I was asleep.

Next to my bed I found a note from Barbara, Ralph's wife. The service was at 1:00 p.m. at Grandville's Northwest Chapel. The burial would be private, thankfully. The thought of visiting a cemetery and watching as Ralph was lowered into the ground would send me over the edge. Just seeing him in a coffin would be enough for me. Another note, this one from Henry, informed me he was picking me up at 11:30 a.m., so we had plenty of time to get there and get a good seat. According to Nurse Hadley, the font of information while taking my vitals, I was the only Shady Valley resident who was attending. Out of the five of us left who had known Ralph, I was the only one considered ambulatory.

I decided to wear my pink sweat suit. It always made Ralph smile. Henry arrived to pick me up wearing an ink-colored suit and a somber tie. Very un-Henry. "Are you sure you're allowed to wear pink to this?" Henry asked. "I thought you were supposed to be in black."

"I promised Ralph I'd wear this to his service. He told me I'd give him someone to smile with since everybody else would look like you," I answered. Henry and I seemed to be blessed with an easy peace between us, at least for now. For this day.

We brought my wheelchair to ensure a good seat, no matter how late we were. We weren't late, though, and as he wheeled me in, parting the seas of people with his "excuse us" and "pardon us," I felt eyes looking at me and quickly looking away. At last I saw Barbara and the kids.

"Oh Jenn, I'm so glad you're here. You wore Ralph's favorite color. How thoughtful," she said, bending down to give me a hug. She and Henry hugged.

"Your friend, the short fellow, he's here, inside the chapel," Barbara said before turning to hug the next person in line. That'd be Henry's job someday. Better him than me. Even if I beat this thing—when I beat this thing—and we're both ninety-nine and ready, I wanted to die first. I never wanted to be the one left behind to hug.

Jacob, "the short fellow," sat on the aisle in the front row of folding seats. Henry moved a chair, parked me next to Jacob, and sat next to me. As I held hands with both of them, I found the nerve to look up. The coffin was mahogany with an elegant sheen, lined in white satin. I'm sure it came with a matching satin pillow. Ralph's hands were crossed on his chest in that death pose, and under his crossed hands was a book. The Bible, I supposed.

"I've already gone for the viewing, but I can help if you'd like," Jacob whispered.

"I don't know if I can handle it," I said.

"You should, Jenn. Plus, I want to know what he's holding in his hand," Jacob whispered. "It's not a Bible."

Jacob was calm. I knew dozens of his friends and acquaintances had died of AIDS over the years. He was an expert at funerals.

"OK, let's go," I whispered back and squeezed Henry's hand. He'd been silent. The three of us stood together and walked to the line at the casket. If only half of these people would've visited him at Shady Valley, he could've held on longer. Held on to the hope longer. *Where were they when he needed them?* I thought. *Where was I when he needed me? Alone, with Alex.*

People don't look good dead. I remember going to one of my best friend's funerals in high school. She'd been drinking and driving, crashed and died. Her body was displayed in an open casket too. She was pasty, porcelain, dollish. Ralph was too. Too perfect. Too unrumpled. His mannequin hands were draped across *Harvest Time in the Wine Country*.

"Enjoy your visit. I already miss you too much to stay in the valley. I'm going home," I whisper-cried as a tear dropped on Ralph's waxy hands. Henry and Jacob carried me back to our spot, the service began, and then it was over. Jacob went back to Clothes the Loop. Henry and I headed back to Shady Valley, forever without Ralph. I slept the entire ride back, waking up only as Henry carried me into my room and tucked me in.

I woke up mumbling, "It was a stupid mistake. A way to escape from now. Not you and the kids, just the cancer and the treatments. Back to the past, when I was healthy. Alex and I were best friends back then. I trusted him. I didn't have any reason not to."

Henry was in the chair next to the throne. "Trusted your old boyfriend to take you out on a date? Yeah, well, I'm sure you did," he said, oozing anger and sarcasm.

Startled that Henry was there with me, and at his tone, I managed to stammer, "I'm so sorry, Henry." I wasn't good at saying sorry. I never had been. I figured this would be a good time to start improving. No point in hoarding for a later date, given the circumstances. *Hell, pull out the stops,* I told myself.

"Yeah, well, sorry really helps. Shit. I'm sorry too, Jennifer. Don't you think I've been lonely too? Don't you think I'd like to escape sometimes myself? Yes, life has been such a huge walk in the park since this fucking cancer hit us. And yes, I mean us. I've gotten to be a single parent to two young kids, trying to keep focused on my career, trying to take care of you, trying to keep our whole life together. It's not easy from this side either, Jenn. I mean, I'm sorry if he hurt you—if that's what happened—but you had no business going with him in the first place! You're married to me, goddammit!" He had turned his face away from me.

"What do you mean, 'if that's what happened'?" I asked.

"I just want the truth, OK? It's eating me up inside. I want to believe you, but you had a lot of stuff with you, Jennifer. You're saying you were just going to dinner, and he turned psycho, right? Did I get that right?"

"Yes," I said. It sounded more like a croak. My throat was closing as the gap between the truth and a lie sucked the words away. There wasn't any way to explain why Alex packed a bag. I didn't even know why. Nothing made sense, and maybe it never had.

"But why did you pack a suitcase? With enough clothes for a week? You're telling me you weren't planning a romantic getaway or something? That Alex did it against your will, before he took you away. Is that it? You were completely innocent in the whole thing?

"I know how it seems, Henry. I am so sorry. I didn't pack that suitcase, you have to believe me." The tears had started.

"See why I can't believe your bullshit? I tried, but I just can't," Henry said, shifting positions. I noticed it was dark outside and wondered how long he had been sitting there, next to the throne, watching me. Since Ralph's funeral? "At least tell me *why* you did it, Jennifer," Henry said, his voice deadly calm, without inflection. "Why? Am I not enough for you? Do you regret your choice?"

"Henry, of course not. I told you, I love you. I'm a fuckup. Please forgive me," I said, while managing to work my way up to sitting. The room swirled but then settled.

"What does he have that I don't?" he shot back, and I remembered Alex asking that same question not long ago. If only I hadn't gone with Alex. "I've tried to be there for you, for our family, Jennifer. Don't you think there are plenty of women willing, wanting even, to comfort me these last few months?"

My head shot up at this last bit, and I looked at him closely. Did he have a confession of his own? I held my breath and waited.

"How do you think it makes me feel, resisting temptation, standing beside you all this time, then knowing that the minute I leave town for a couple of days, you hop in the car to go God knows where with your old boyfriend? Why am I not enough?"

"It was a mistake. Trusting him. I love you, not him," I said, forcing the words out between sobs. "He hurt me, and I didn't want him to. You have to believe that. I didn't mean for it to happen. I can't lose you. Us."

Henry turned on the chair, and we were face to face. The anger inside him rose like steam, charging the air between us. His voice was no longer in control.

"A trusted friend you let take you to a deserted lake house? Come on, I'm not stupid. Tell me the rest."

"Can we get past this?" I asked.

"I really don't know yet," he said, his back to me again. "I want to know everything that happened. From the beginning."

The story, once minimized to its base elements, was clear-cut, at least to me. I spared Henry the rekindled desire I felt every time Alex visited at Shady Valley. He already suspected that, anyway.

"I was alone and feeling sorry for myself, and Alex offered an escape. For some reason, I didn't know he was obsessed with me until we were having dinner, and it was too late. I thought he was dating Julie and that we could be just friends, friends having dinner," I added. But could I tell Henry that it felt so good to be wanted, to be worshipped even? To have romantic surprises brought to me at Shady Valley? To have the freedom of not worrying, of not thinking of anything other than what I wanted right then? And what I wanted right then was out of there. Away from the sterile world and back to a dream world of passion, when anything was possible and I was young and alive. Away from a place where my best friend was dying. No, I couldn't say all of that, so I simply said, "Things got scary and he lost control. Finally, I talked him into taking me back."

Simple. Stupid. Sneaky. Bad.

"Let me see the bruises, Jennifer," he said.

That was the moment when time stopped. The moment of proof. There was no denying anything now.

I pulled the sheet down to my waist and pulled my sweatshirt up over my face. My bare arms were illuminated by the Shady Valley institutional glow, revealing the evidence he sought. A handprint on my right upper arm. Bruises encircling my left. I hoped that would be enough.

"Oh my god. The bastard," Henry said quietly as I sat on the throne allowing him to examine me. "We're pressing charges. Oh my god, we're pressing charges. How could this happen? How could you let this happen? Did you sleep with him? Where is he now? I'm going to kill him."

"No," I said, shivering, gurgling sounds coming from my mouth, not knowing what to say, what to do. I wrapped my shirt back around me, but it didn't help. As Henry walked toward the door, away from me, I called, "No! Henry, please, come back. I'm so sorry. It's OK now. I'm OK now. Please." I knew this was it. The time when he would decide. My husband could, at any moment, walk away. No more caring for invalids. No more single parenting. Just leave. Find someone young, and healthy, and normal. There were plenty. He said so himself. Somebody faithful. Somebody good. Not deceitful. For the first time in my illness, in my life, I was completely alone.

14

Warning: Potential shock hazard.

A LITTLE WHILE AFTER HENRY LEFT, MY FAVORITE DOCTOR OF the bunch, Mary Butcher, waltzed in, her heels tap-tap-tapping on the fake-wood floor. Mary was my internal medicine doctor, from the days when all I complained about were winter sinus infections. Although she didn't have to diagnose the cancer, since I was still under the care of my OB, Mary had been by my side ever since. *I wonder if I remembered to invite her to my party. I wonder if I still need a party.*

"I've wanted to come by for two weeks, and I just said, 'I'm going today, no matter what.' How are you doing? Am I interrupting anything?" she asked.

"No, of course not. It's wonderful to see you," I said, happy for the distraction. I didn't know if Henry ever would be back. Ralph was dead. I was alone.

"How are you doing?" Mary perched on the edge of my bed, leaning close to me, to my face. Her perky brown hair was held back by the reading glasses she only donned to write prescriptions. Her white doctor's coat had just the faintest of stains, showing a long day at the office. The white coat covered a two-piece, dark-green St. John knit suit that looked immaculate. Her eyes, like a fawn's, were intense and soft at the same time.

She broke the dam with that look. I couldn't speak. In fact, I could barely breathe. I was crying in big, body-shaking gasps.

Mary sat, doe eyes caring, her hand patting mine in a half-friend, half-mom action. "It's good to let it out," she said. "You know, I think they'd like to kick you out of here soon. I've talked to your team—there are some new options, some new experimental drugs and gene therapy treatments. I'll help sort through the options, when you're up to it."

Finally, when I'd calmed down enough to listen, she spoke. "Listen, Jenn. Listen. People diagnosed with a serious, perhaps terminal, disease often suffer from post-traumatic stress disorder. I know that sounds strange, as you aren't post-disease—yet—but the point is that what you're suffering from is normal. To doubt everything in your life, to want outside validation, to want to hold on to what was good in the past, that's normal. Please know that," she said.

I looked into her kind eyes. I wanted to believe I was OK. I was worth saving, just as I knew our marriage was worth saving. The tears rolled down my cheeks, but I was listening.

"We also know that there is a phenomenon called post-traumatic growth; the positive aspect of a dire health condition includes a greater sense of personal strength, a renewed appreciation of life, spirituality, and closeness with others. But, really, all of this is secondary to getting past what happened to you with that old boyfriend, because, as you may suspect by now, that is another major trauma—suffering physical violence. Oh, and the death of a friend," she said. She'd seen my files—of course she had. "You've been through a lot, girlfriend. But let's realize things are looking up."

My tears stopped as my brain worked to process everything I was learning. "So I've turned the corner?" I asked.

"Yes, I think so. Honey, you have a great marriage, two wonderful kids, parents who love you, a host of friends who are swarming into town to see you. I'd say you're blessed. I'd say not only does God love you, but a lot of people do too. And, like I told you and you seemed to ignore, you've been accepted into a new trial, and you can do this treatment at home."

Home, I thought. The concept was hard to believe. I tried to remember the baby-powder smell of our home, the sounds of my children laughing, the colors of my garden. "You are the best," I said, reaching up to give Mary a hug.

"You are. This was the best part of my day. You're going to beat this. I know it."

"Did I invite you to my going-away party?" I asked.

"Yes, and I'd be glad to come. I hope I don't need a date, because I won't have one. By the way, where are you going?" Mary asked.

"I'm not sure," I answered.

Looking at the row of pill bottles on my bureau, I thought, *People should come with warning labels.* Somewhere on your back, God would print a list of ingredients: generous, hardworking, musical, and the rest of the good, along with a list of harmful ingredients: jealous, lazy, drug addled, narcissistic, dreamer. Below the ingredients would be a scale representing potential to change. And finally, a calorie count. How much would this person weigh in your life? Would you have to carry him like a child all through life? Or was he too light, too much in the clouds to live in the real world? Would 50 percent of all people in the United States divorce if we knew what the other person was made of going in? No way—you could dump the loser recipes right away. If you read, "potential to leave in midlife and marry a secretarial bimbo," he'd be gone. "Will beat you and then bring you roses,"—I don't think so.

Henry's ingredients were character, love, and strength. How could I have doubted his love for me? It was because I'd doubted myself, I supposed. If you don't feel worthy of love, if something is missing, or something horrible is thrust upon you, it's easy to doubt your worth. And it's even easier for someone with skill to take advantage of that weakness.

What would Alex's label be? Duplicitous, scheming, liar. No, not really. I loved him once, and he was better than he was that night at the lake. I had missed the warning signs that something wasn't right with him. That he was unhappy. Two unhappy people trying to find something reflected in each other, tied together by the past.

If I hadn't lost faith in myself, in the life I'd created with Henry, Alex would have been no more than another visitor. If I had explained to Henry that I needed attention as his wife, as a woman, I could have found everything I needed with the man who visited me whenever I called.

"Jennifer, honey," Daddy said as he walked into my room.

"I thought you were golfing," I said, surprised and delighted by his surprise visit.

"Ah, that's what I told your mother to get away from her," he said, giving me a big hug and settling in on the end of the throne. "I love you so much, Jennifer. Your doctors said they are going to let you go home. I am—well, you were always my favorite. My little girl is going home."

"Yes, Daddy, I know," I said. My cheeks were already so numb from tears I could barely feel them trickle. I didn't care. "But you never visit me here, just one time this whole month. And I thought about you all the time. In my dreams you were there, a picture-perfect daddy. By my bedside, challenging the doctors, playing Monopoly with me," I said.

"You always beat me at Monopoly. I'd never play *that* game with you," he said.

"Just hide and seek. That's all we've been playing. You're always hiding, and I'm always seeking," I said, knowing it was hurting both of us to talk like this. But I had to be honest.

"This has been the most difficult thing in my life, watching you suffer." A tear rolled down his left cheek. I reached up and wiped it with my tissue. I reached over and held his hand.

"I'm getting better," I said.

"Do you think I've been there for you?" he asked.

"I know you think about me, and the weekly flowers are great, but I guess I'm talking about time. Just time spent. Like a date. I didn't know I had so much competition, Henry, the golf course, whatever," I said.

"Let's make a plan. You get out of here, and we'll take a trip, just the two of us, to some exciting place, and spend lots of money and eat out and talk. I'll even let you beat me in Monopoly, as usual," Daddy said, his dry hand squeezing mine.

"Let me?" I asked. "It's a plan. After the party on Friday, I don't have a lot going on. Did you know Ralph died?"

"I know, honey, but don't let it scare you—he had a totally different disease. Wonderful man, though. You're going to beat this, Jennifer. Dr. Chris is optimistic about the new treatment, and so am I. I think it's time for you to go home to your family and recover there. Henry misses you," Daddy said. "He's a fine young man. Perfect for the succession plan. He'll need help if I'm not around, and you have the best business mind in the family. You take after me."

"Thanks, Daddy," I said.

"Oh, and honey, do try to be patient with your mother. I know she's taxing. God knows. But she's so dependent, so helpless. She's just—"

"Heavy?" I asked.

"I guess that's a good way to describe it. I dreamed of a wonderful, blessed marriage. That's really what I wanted. And I married a princess. Me. A Hollywood star said yes to me—that's what I thought at the time," he said as he squeezed my hand. "You're the positive outcome, Jennifer. You're the light in my life."

And Juliana's the mother of your children. And Julie's just a miniature version of Juliana, Juliana as child. If only it were so simple. If only it weren't so true. "Is Julie still in town, Daddy?" I asked, wondering how much he knew about Julie and Alex—how much there was to know.

"Far as I know, she is, honey, though I don't see her much. She and your mom, well they're thick as thieves," he answered. "I do love those little girls of hers."

I smiled and patted his hand. He'd checked out of his own house long ago. Whatever Julie was up to, she had free reign of our family home and more.

"Well, I'm going to head out, honey," Dad said, kissing me on the cheek. "I'll be by for your party, I suppose, but after that it's all about healing."

15

**Warning: Women with a history of depression
should be carefully observed.**

SUNSHINE WAS STREAMING IN THROUGH MY WINDOW, AND HADLEY
was placing a tray of nondescript food on my bedside table. "Morning,"
she said, nodding, smile-free, before exiting.

Dr. Mary called and babbled on and on about the new therapy.
"This will be the one," she said. As my primary care doctor, she was
the quarterback of my team and the cheerleader. She had called
a meeting of all my specialists and their subspecialists. *Go team,* I
thought drearily. It was nice, but I had heard it. I wasn't hopeless—
just realistic and tired. *Maybe she was right about post-traumatic
stress disorder.*

Dr. Mary had told me the symptoms of PTSD were depression
and anxiety, vivid flashbacks, emotional detachment—all symptoms I
experienced. Knowing that what I was feeling had a name was a relief.

And I knew what I needed to do to get better. I needed to go home.

"Then you should. That's what you should do. You're stable enough
to go," Nurse Hadley said walking back into the room. Where had
she come from? How did she hear me?

"What about my party? I'm having it here," I said.

"Move it to your home. I'm sure your friends will help make calls, notify everybody in time. I think you're right. You should go home," she said. "It'd be best for everyone. I'll come and take care of you there, if you'd like."

"Um, OK," I said. "Will you talk to the staff physician, tell him to call Henry? See if I can get out of here tomorrow, if possible. Please? Just don't pull rank on him, Hadley."

I had to go home. Be with the kids. My talk with Dr. Mary had clarified everything. I was tired of living in a bubble. Despite my new hopes, I couldn't escape the feeling that I was running out of time. Besides, I was stabilized. We could have a full-time nurse, someone like Nurse Mary Ann or Nurse Samuels. Not Nurse Hadley, unless I got sicker again. We could call the guests and just move my party home.

Home. That used to mean my parents' house. I could still hear Julie banging on the grand piano, supposedly practicing her scales. And I remembered the piano man's warning the day he delivered it. He said, "That piano, like a person, needs time to settle into a new home." He would give our piano two months and return to tune it again.

Home. College. Great friends. My first apartment.

Home. My early twenties. Finding myself, finishing with Alex, being alone for the first time.

Home. Henry. I'd been lucky enough to live the dream, even if only for a short while. A loving husband, a beautiful home, a successful business, and beautiful children. I needed to go home again.

But first, I had to say good-bye to my best friend at Shady Valley.

My heart thumped as I walked down the hall to Ralph's room. His door was closed, but I opened it and went in. Ralph's smell was still here—his Old Spice cologne—and I had to move quickly to sit in one of his burgundy chairs. The bed was unmade, but someone had tidied up the room. It was as if Ralph had just popped out for a walk and would be back any moment to climb back onto his throne.

His reading glasses were on the bedside table, and our Scrabble game box was on the bottom shelf.

"Ralph, why did you leave me?" I asked, dropping my head into my hands. "I am so sorry I wasn't here for you when you needed me. I could've kept holding on. I know I would've pulled you back here, back to us, if I hadn't been so stupid, so selfish. I'm so sorry, Ralph."

I stood up and made my way slowly to his bed, sitting down on it and clasping his readers in my left hand. "How did I let my best friend in the world down? How could you die when I was away? Did you know how wrong I was to leave? Did you call for me? No one will tell me. Oh Ralph, please forgive me. Please, please, forgive me.

"There really is no excuse that I can give you, but I sort of left here with Alex, because I was jealous that you had a date, and Henry and Dad were golfing, and you got sick, and it turned out terrible. But now Henry and I are talking and fighting—and I think we'll end up in a better place. I've missed talking to you so much, through all of this, but then you had to go and die just when I needed you. Well, I've always needed you here," I said. "That's why I'm going home." I lay back against Ralph's cold pillow, and I thought back to our relationship, from friendship to flirting when both of us were feeling the same neglect from our spouses and isolation within the walls of Shady Valley. Circumstances brought us together—similar fates—but our kindred spirits allowed us to develop a close friendship. I was so glad we never crossed that line, except for one kiss. It would have ruined us. Pure friendship, pure love. I'd never find this type of accelerated, intensified friendship again—I knew it.

"Oh Ralph, please, forgive me. I love you, forgive me, rest in peace, my friend," I said climbing out of his bed. I took one last look around his room and walked out the door, his readers grasped in my left hand.

I was to be discharged in the morning, but I hadn't heard from Henry since our fight. Paige called and let me know the hospital bed had arrived at home and that the kids were overjoyed at my homecoming. Obviously, Henry had made the arrangements. But what else was he doing? Had he found Alex? Confronted him? Had he gone to the police? I'd checked my cell phone repeatedly, and my texts to his phone went unanswered.

I couldn't go home, be home, unless Henry wanted me there. I sat on the throne, holding Ralph's readers, and wondered what to do. I realized there was nothing I could do. As Henry had said, I'd done enough. Now it was Henry's move. I said a little prayer for God's forgiveness and Henry's, and turned on the news.

I'd watched at least four half-hour segments when there was a knock on my door.

"Come in," I said, hoping, praying it was my husband.

It was.

Henry was dressed in my favorite blue jeans and a long-sleeved white T-shirt. He looked relaxed and happy—a far different man than the one who left my room in anger just two days earlier.

"Hey, Jenn," he said as he pulled a bunch of white Gerbera daisies from behind his back and handed them to me. A peace offering, I hoped.

"Hey, Henry, they're beautiful," I said, clicking off the news and waiting for his next move.

After he put the daisies in water, he pulled up the brown chair next to the throne and sat down. It was as if we were having a meeting. I waited.

"Jennifer. I need to know, did he rape you?"

I shook my head. "No, it stopped. He stopped," I said before lowering my eyes, breaking our gaze.

Henry was silent for moment, and then said, "Shit. Shit. Shit."

"Henry, please. What's the point? It's over. We don't have the time. We need to move past this, past him. He only ruins our life together if we keep him in it." My stomach had worked itself into knots so tight I thought I'd be sick. My heart raced. "Don't let him break us apart. That's what he wants."

"He's done a great job making his wishes come true." Henry picked up the remote control to the television, and I thought he was going to turn it on. Instead, he looked at me intently and said, "He's a bastard."

"He only wins if you let him." Now I was pleading. For our life.

"I can't believe you've covered for him. Hiding this, these—from me," he said, rubbing his fingers down the outside of my right arm. The bruise flamed through the sweatshirt I had on. "Didn't you think I deserved to know about it, bruises and all?"

"I wasn't covering for him. This is all my fault, my fault he hurt me, and I didn't want him to hurt you, too. That's why I didn't show you. Don't you see what it's done to you? The knowing?"

We sat side by side, sort of, him on the brown chair, me on the throne. Both of us stared out my window, outside to the real world beyond Shady Valley. I'd try to look at him, meet his eyes with mine, but he wouldn't turn toward me.

"Do you still love him?" he finally asked.

I forced a laugh. Was he kidding? "No. I love you. Always have. Always will. I am so sorry." I lay back then on the throne, crying quietly. I turned onto my side, away from him. Away from the husband I'd hurt too deeply to fix. After another eternity, I felt his body curling up, fitting in behind me on the bed.

"I'll try, Jennifer, to get over this," he whispered.

"Thank you," I said, rolling over on my back to embrace him. His tears dropped onto my face, causing a blink and a mutual chuckle. It felt good to smile, even a little.

"Eventually I will have to deal with Alex in my own way, you know. But for now, we'll keep him out of our life."

I felt a wave of relief, like I'd been to the brink and back. Because of one wrong decision, I had almost lost everything. But now, having

Henry here with me, on my bed, I felt saved and safe. I sank into an exhausted, merciful sleep.

The next thing I knew, I awoke to golden light streaming in across the bed. Even more unfamiliar was the profile of my sleeping husband beside me. For the first time in months—fifteen months to be exact, from the time of my diagnosis—I felt lucky. No matter what. The last two years had been lost in a sea of morning sickness, labor, delivery, surgery, radiation, chemo, and lately, experimental immunotherapies and gene therapy. I was alive and in love. Most important, I had been given a second chance.

"Henry, I love you," I said, reaching my arm across his chest and squeezing him. It had been so long since we shared the same bed, without IV tubes, newborns, sickness between us.

"Morning. I love you too," he murmured sleepily.

I snuggled in closer to him and listened to the steady pounding of his heart. I wanted that heart to be strong and not broken, not destroyed forever by what I had done. I hoped we could both start healing, together. I knew it would take time. I hoped I had enough. At least he was willing to try.

"We need to get packing. It's time to go home," Henry said.

"OK. Let's do it," I answered. I'd never felt more lucky in my life. "Henry, do you think we can go to the pumpkin fields when we get home? It has to be almost pumpkin time, and Hannah didn't get to go last year, and I know you took Hank, but I want the four of us to go."

"That's a great idea," Henry answered, wrestling a large blue suitcase down from the top of my closet. "This is the suitcase *he* packed for you, in case you didn't know."

"I didn't. I told you that," I said, busying myself in my bathroom.

"Jennifer, tell me this," Henry said, "Did you think you still loved him? Is that why you left with him?"

So much for the peaceful packing moment. I sighed and walked out of the bathroom. "Not love like our love. But I guess, for the love I had with him, back then, yes, I guess I thought I still loved him. I thought I still knew him. Obviously, on both counts, I was so wrong. I can't tell you sorry enough," I answered as honestly as possible.

"I've thought about it, and I realized how preoccupied I've been lately. I've been so caught up in my own world—I haven't really been there for you, have I? Our date nights are really just me complaining about work or the kids or whatever. I'm sorry too."

"Henry, you've been amazing. Taking care of me. With the kids. You're everything I ever wanted. I'm the one who screwed up. I was lonely and feeling sorry for myself. You and Daddy got to leave town, have fun. Julie is back in town and living life. Ralph and Barb were off on a date. Suddenly, Alex was there, giving me attention. I was selfish and childish. He treated me like the person I used to be. Not a sick person, not a mom—a woman. When Ralph got so sick…It was stupid. I just want us to get past it, while we still can," I said. I sat down on the throne and cried.

Shockingly, Henry sat down beside me and started crying too. And we sat there, truly side by side, hoping nobody appeared at the door.

"I hate it when I do this," Henry said, wiping his eyes self-consciously. "I feel like a fern."

"A fern? What do you mean you feel like a fern?" I asked.

"You know, all moist, and drippy, and stuff," he said, beginning to smile.

I couldn't help it—I burst out laughing. Henry joined in, and we were laugh-crying. Together.

When we'd finally stopped laughing, I asked, "Do you think all marriages, after a while, get to be just friendships? Or worse? Is the 'better' all gone by the early stages?"

"I hope not, Jenn," Henry said, looking into my eyes. "I think it depends on the people involved, how much they're willing to fight for the relationship, and how much they let come between them."

"Like old boyfriends," I said, looking down at my hands, the pain of guilt clinching my stomach.

"Or work, or kids, or a serious illness, or financial troubles," Henry said. "Hey, you aren't the only one who is to blame, I realize that now. I do. I was here physically but not emotionally."

"Thank you, Henry," I said. "Have you been talking to someone about this, about us?"

"Let's just say Pastor Barker has helped me see the light," Henry said, before standing up.

God bless Pastor Barker, I thought as I fell into my husband's warm embrace.

"And now, let's get packing. I know two little kids who can't wait to see their mommy back home," Henry said.

I stared into Henry's eyes, misted with tears. "I'm going home," I said before bursting into tears again.

16

Warning: To prevent injury, do not disassemble.

At home I got to hug my babies and have them sleep with me. We'd nap together, and I could help give them baths. We could watch Barney. And read. And play with toys. Being home with Henry and the kids made my heart sing.

Once I was back, I couldn't believe I had been able to withstand being away for so long. Why hadn't I insisted on going home sooner? For one thing, I had been too weak to even get up and go to the bathroom alone during my first weeks at Shady Valley, I reminded myself. Recently I had felt better than I had in months. Being back at home was providing some sort of new energy surge too, and I hoped it lasted.

Outside the window, the morning sun was turning the clouds orange. That was a good sign: orange is the color of happiness. All my friends were coming to town. I was home, surrounded by my own things for the first time in months. How easy was it to take all of this—home and my family—for granted before I was sick? How easy was it to dismiss Henry and our love when I was feeling my worst? I had almost ruined everything for a night of escapism. I shuddered.

I indulged myself with the thought of last night's reunion. "Mommy's here! Mommy's home," Hank had yelled from the open front door as Henry and I made our way up the walk. How I wished I had my camera out to capture the look on his face: pure, innocent joy, with love on top.

"Come give me a big squeeze, Hankster!" I yelled back, and he charged, all thirty-one pounds of bouncy blond baby racing down the walkway and smashing into me. He would've knocked me over if Henry hadn't steadied me from behind. I squatted down next to him, kissing him and rubbing my fingers along his soft, perfect arms.

"I've missed you, so much," I said.

"Pick up me," Hank demanded.

"I'll get you, champ. Mommy's not quite strong enough yet. But she'll hold you on her lap and rock you, if you'd like," Henry said, scooping him up and still holding me.

"Yeaaaah!" Hank yelled. He remained exuberant for hours. As Henry and the moving company he'd hired tried to squeeze my stuff—clothes, supplies, equipment—into what used to be Henry's office, Hank was busy talking to a moving man, drawing me a picture, sitting on my lap. Hannah watched the chaos, not talking, just observing and every once in a while letting out a squeal. When she did, Hank said, "That hurts my ears. No, no, Haywa."

I couldn't wait until she and I could go on buying trips together. She could help me stay current, keep the Loop on top. It would be so much fun. We had so much to do, Hannah and me—all of us, as a family. I had to be there for it. I had to.

When Jacob walked in, interrupting my reverie, I said, "That is so funny—I was just thinking about the Loop. How Hannah could help keep us current, you know, as she grows up and we grow old."

"Welcome home. I love what you've done with the office," he joked and handed me the usual bunch of daisies.

"You don't have to bring me flowers every visit, you know," I said. "So tell me about another record-breaking week at the store."

"I'd like to, but with back to school, a lot of our customers are busy buying kids' clothes and school supplies. It drops off at the end of summer. Always," Jacob said. "Don't worry. As soon as those kids have been back in school for a bit, we'll see a big bump. Also, temperatures will drop, and they'll think of football and fall clothes. It's clockwork." Then he asked, "Any problems settling in?"

"I just hope I can fit back in—literally and figuratively," I said, looking around the room. Henry's office, before all this, had been a bastion of male tranquility. Dark wood walls, dark wood floors, oriental carpet, and a really neat half-moon desk we'd found at an antique store in Chicago. Now it was a hospital room, complete with hospital bed, IV stand, and all the other medical equipment I needed, plus my television, telephone, and computer, and a dresser I could reach from the bed to hold all the things I grabbed on a regular basis.

The office was in the southwest corner of the first floor and was flooded by bright sunshine. I would need to get accustomed to light again.

"I just wanted you to know your fridge is stocked and ready for any and all visitors, and the party is on track for Friday, here," Jacob said. "I just thought since your mom is a little, um, stressed out, it would be OK if I handled the details. I really think it's going to be so much nicer at your home. More intimate, you know?"

"Thank you, Jacob. I will make it up to you, you know. I promise. You're the best."

"Make it up to me by getting better, Jennifer—promise?" He turned on his two-inch platform shoes and left before either of us had a chance to cry.

The cleaning lady Henry hired was terrific: quiet, efficient, and good. Before her, we employed a woman who believed cancer was contagious. She quit after hearing my diagnosis. Some people were like that, believing they could catch cancer like a cold. I could sense those people now. They air-kissed your cheek and stood as far away as possible without being obviously rude. I scared them, either physically, because they thought I'd infect them, or mentally, because they couldn't handle the reality of death. I was a reminder: just look at the sickle-shaped shadows under my eyes.

After the cleaning lady left, and before naptime, we had a picnic in Mommy's Room, as it was currently dubbed. Paige, Hank, Hannah, and me.

Soon after the kids went down, I spotted company walking up the front path. From my perch on my new throne, a truer throne, with the blinds pulled half-way down, all I could see as visitors approached the front door were the bottom half of people's bodies, mostly just legs and feet. I guessed, from the legs, that Betsy—in a cute, white skirt and nude pumps—had arrived. "Paige, I'm awake," I said. "You can send her in," I added just as the doorbell rang.

I was right. Betsy, with her bouncy smile and dimples, burst into my room. "Finally, I've got you all to myself," she said, quickly reaching my bed and kissing me on the forehead. "This is much better, seeing you here. At home. You even look better." Betsy's brunette bob and brown eyes shined, and her smile was infectious.

"What do you think of the suit?" she asked, twirling on her high heels, and I realized she was sporting a two-piece summer-white knit from my store.

"It's perfect on you. I'm so glad you guys went by the Loop. Did you tell Jacob who you were?" I asked, hoping Jacob didn't jabber at her too much.

"No, actually, but he's a trip—no wonder you guys get along so well." Betsy laughed.

"Here's a question for you: if you could go back to college, start all over again, would you do it? If not, is there another period of life you'd go back to?"

"I'd go back to college in a flash," Betsy answered. "I loved it there. Talking. Thinking. Dreaming. But, no, what am I saying? I'd stay right where I am," she said, echoing my own sentiments. "This is the best time of life. My kids are great. I love Mike. I love my workouts and my friends and the Junior League. Some might think I lead a shallow life, but it's more depth than I've ever felt, more full."

"I'd stay too, without cancer," I said. It was funny, though—a few weeks ago, I would have said I'd like to return to college, or high school even, to escape the present, to escape the lack of emotional connection in my marriage, to escape the cancer. Did the cancer cause Henry and me to grow apart or had life, in general, done that? Were we just going through the motions of a relationship while we focused on raising the kids and growing our separate businesses? I wondered what would have happened to my marriage without Alex. Without someone else coming into the relationship and making me feel alive again. Even without cancer, I would have answered the question by saying I'd return to college. How selfish. How escapist. What I needed to do was confront Henry in the present, instead of dreaming about the past. I needed to let him know what I was feeling and thinking, what I was missing in our relationship, instead of kissing the first other man who showed an interest in me.

How easily I was distracted by Alex and lost sight of what was important. Thank God there was still time.

"Speaking of staying, Henry informed me visitation is one hour, tops, because you need to get your strength back before the big party. I'm heading over to your mother's house, to pick up all the party supplies and confirm numbers with the caterer," Betsy said. "Is there anything you need?'

"Not with friends like you. Thanks," I said, blessed by all the attention. "Have you run into Liza or Wendy? They are in town for the party and said they'd help if we needed them."

"I think I have everything covered. Take a nap now, so you can play with the kids when they wake up," she added while hustling out of the room, a blur of white.

Henry knocked, self-consciously, and blushed before walking straight to me and wrapping me in a huge embrace.

"Wow, what is that for?" I asked, breathing him in.

"For being home," he answered. "This is the best. I'm so much happier; the kids are so much happier. This final drug is going to work, and we are going to get back to normal, Jenn. Hell, better than normal."

"I'm game," I said, kissing him deeply. "And thank you, again, for taking me back, for your forgiveness." I hoped we were finished fighting. I believed he hoped for that too.

"Of course, honey," Henry answered. "Now get some sleep. We've got a busy couple of days coming up, thanks to this crazy party of yours," Henry said as he shuffled away to figure out dinner for the kids.

I was still groggy from the emotional scene and the following nap when Juliana arrived. The sun, once so bright in my office bed-room, was gone from most of my windows.

"Mother?" I said to the shadow in the doorway. I knew it was her; it smelled like her. She shouldn't plan to sneak up on anyone, not when she was wearing Oscar.

"Yes, dear, are you asleep?" Mother asked, sitting down on a mid-night-blue, oversized chair near the window. In the moment before she sat, I saw in the light that she was wearing her navy Channel suit, her navy hosiery, and Ferragamo pumps. The chair swallowed her: all I could see from my bed was her bright-red mouth.

"No, I'm awake. How are you?"

"How are *you*?" she asked.

Ah, there it was. Concern for her sick daughter had emerged and at last been articulated. *Be nice,* I reminded myself. She was still smiling, red lips, white teeth. I was talking to a big-mouthed chair.

"I'm feeling great, so much better. Where has Julie been?" I asked, trying to sound breezy.

"I expect her to be visiting you anytime now," Mother answered, sounding mysterious.

"What do you mean 'anytime now'?" I asked.

The blue chair had no comment. Then Juliana sighed. A deep, dramatic gesture that counterintuitively sucked the air out of the room. "You should feel sorry for Julie. She isn't as lucky in love as you are," Mother said finally.

Lucky? I thought about how close I had come to losing Henry already. We had only been married six years. Who was I to judge, to condemn my parents' relationship, or my sister's? Marriage was tough. "Henry and I have faced one of the toughest things a relationship can face—a terminal illness. I would be lucky if I were here, alive, in thirty years and still married to Henry. But I think it takes work. You know that. It's not luck. You and Daddy have been together thirty-five years, most of them blissful."

"Ha," she said, a snorting sound that became another sigh. She sounded like the lead goose in the *V*. "Keep your head down and flap. This is how things are supposed to be." So cynical.

"So, when did you stop loving him?" I asked her.

"Why, Jennifer, never. I've loved your father since the day I saw him. At that party in La Jolla. I thought he was in the movie industry. It was love at first sight. I mean, the fact I thought he was a producer just added to it. We went on a date. He told me he had to leave in the morning—for Ohio. Ohio? But I liked him. He treated me like a star. I wasn't one. But by the time we married, I was a star. To him. To everyone in Grandville."

"So, it's a wonderful life?" I asked, tears springing to my eyes.

"It's a wonderful life, Jennifer," she said. "Oh baby, look at you. All your friends in town, and now your face will be a mess." Mother crossed the room and wiped my cheeks with a tissue she magically produced out of thin air. A definite mom trick—I would have to learn that one. "Shhh, sweetie, you're home now, and you're getting better. Everything will be wonderful," she added, reaching for my hand.

At last, her perfectly made-up mask dissolved before my eyes and tears streaked her cheeks with the dark stains of many coats of mascara. For the first time in months, maybe years, her arms encircled me in a genuine embrace, and we held each other close for a long time.

At last, Mother sniffed and straightened. She touched my cheek again, lightly. "I'll be OK, you know, as long as you get better. And you will too. You look so much better since you've come home— except for the ruined makeup, of course," she joked weakly. "I'll come early on Friday and help you do your face, OK, dear?"

"Sure, Mother, that'd be great." Our relationship would probably never be deep, but she did try, I knew that now. She gave in the only way she knew how, and she deserved a lot of credit for standing by Daddy all those years. *And I certainly didn't make it any easier on her,* I realized with a sudden pang of remorse.

She patted my hand and straightened her shoulders. Sighing resolutely, Juliana pasted a big smile on her face and rose to leave.

"Your friends have taken over the party planning, Jennifer, and I'm really so relieved. But there are so many last minute details to attend to, you know. Get your beauty sleep, dear—I'll see you Friday!"

And she was off, leaving me wondering when Julie would appear.

16

**Warning: Contains mature content.
May not be suitable for all audiences.**

THE BEST THING ABOUT BEING HOME WAS LISTENING TO THE morning sounds. They were so comforting. I heard Henry in the kitchen starting the coffee and talking, probably to Hank. I could picture Hank wearing feetie pajamas, sucking his pacifier, and resting his head on his dad's shoulder. His eyes would be squeezed shut so that the sun wouldn't "poke him in the eye," as he said. I hoped they would remember me in here. I could protect Hank from the sun.

The doorbell was ringing. I heard Henry walk past my room to answer it. It sounded like it was the nurse. He told her I was asleep, but I wasn't. I heard her voice, and I was glad she was here. Maybe she'd tell me I looked great. That I was saved. That she could tell, from working with the dying all the time, that I'd crossed back over. That I was one of the living.

One of the living who had to worry about gaining weight, about buying the right wardrobe essentials for fall. One of the living who had to worry about home prices falling or holding, about saving for college. Maybe I'd be allowed to care again if the Ohio State Buckeyes beat Iowa this weekend. I mean, dare I care? I could hope, but should I care?

"Hello? Jennifer?" said the friendly-sounding nurse.

"Yep, I'm awake," I answered.

Much to my surprise, Nurse Hadley trotted in. *Hadley? Really?* Hadn't I had enough of her?

"I know, what a surprise I must be," Hadley exclaimed. "Oh, your home is lovely, exquisite, actually. I love the artwork—and those two blue chairs, amazing."

I knew I was staring at her, but Hadley wasn't Hadley. She wore a dark-brown shift dress that accented her curves, brown pumps that were—could they be?—Jimmy Choos. A delicate pearl necklace completed the look.

"Nurse Hadley? What's happened to you?" I stammered.

"Well, we both have our institutional looks and our real-world looks, don't we?" she answered before pulling out her medical bag and beginning the typical vital sign tests. "I have become quite a fan of the Loop, you know."

What? Jacob had never mentioned a word about this. *Traitor.* "Why, I didn't know, but thank you," I said. After she'd poked and prodded, listened and timed, I had to ask: "You haven't said anything about how I look, Nurse Hadley."

"No, no, I haven't," she answered. "I'd say you look fine. Just fine." And with that, she packed up her bag and left.

I could hear Henry and Hadley talking in the hall, but I couldn't discern what they were saying. Was I worse? The same? Better? Now I didn't know.

"Henry!" I called once I had watched Nurse Hadley and her elegant heels maneuver down the front walk.

As he walked in the door I asked, "Do I look better? Do I?"

"Of course. You're here, with us. You're home. Everything is better. You look, sound, taste"—he walked over and kissed me, deeply—"yes, taste better," Henry said. He sat on the bed and took my hand.

"I've been thinking. I realized I've never been more hurt in my life," Henry said. "I can get past it, I will get past it. I'm having trouble getting Alex out of my head. The two of you, together. Making out—even if you didn't have sex, I know more went on. I know you, Jenn. You're trying to protect me."

He looked to me for a response. What more could I say than I had already?

"That said, I'm so happy to have you home, to have all of us under one roof. My happy family, and we will be happy, Jenn," he said.

"Henry, I love you," I said, pulling him down on top of me. The hospital bed was supposed to be a double. I'm not sure how Henry did it, but it seemed to be larger than that. It felt so nice, having the weight of his body on mine. "How did you find such a comfortable bed?" I asked, once he'd rolled over next to me.

"Oh, this. Well, that took a bit of planning," he said. "You know me and beds. You needed comfort, and we needed it to move up and down, just in case, so I had it made. A double-wide. Just for you and me. Oh, and you noticed all the pillows, right?"

"Of course," I said. Henry and his pillows. He could have twenty pillows just for himself and be in heaven. I looked around at Henry, at this bed, this room he made special for me. More than anything I could ever describe or imagine, all of this summed up his love for me. He still wanted to sleep with me—and he made sure we had a bed where I'd be comfortable too.

Indeed, after pulling the shades the rest of the way down, we had complete privacy, and Henry decided it was time for us to try out our new marriage bed.

✳

Betsy and Jacob had called the rest of my book club, and with another of my college roommates, Sam, they called all the guests to inform them about the new party location. Then they started bringing in loads of beautiful flowers, trays of glasses, boxes of candles, the works.

Jacob's partner, Nelson, an auto mechanic normally, took time off to wait on Loop customers and manage our employees so Jacob could be with me. I needed him to be with me. They were great, all of them. Great friends. Great people.

"Remember when we dressed up for that Halloween party as a hot dog?" Sam asked, bringing in a vase of flowers.

"Oh yeah, I forgot about that. You were the little wiener, and Monica and I were the buns. What a great costume." I said.

"I loved those buns," Maddie teased.

"Hey, did I hear somebody talking about my wife's buns?" Henry asked as he walked into the room. He was smiling, and he seemed at ease.

"Not me," Jacob laughed.

"I just wanted you to know, from now on, we have to get together at least once a year, Jennifer. No matter what. When you get stronger, you can come to Nashville, meet my boys in person. Or I'll come here. We need to stay connected. I've missed you. It's easy to forget how much an old friend can mean in your life," Sam said. Her hair was pulled back in a ponytail. She wore yoga pants and a T-shirt from college days. A frat party shirt. Ever since she had arrived, she'd been working hard to get the party set up. They all had.

"That's what this illness has done for me," I said. "It forces you to take stock of all your blessings. That's the main reason I wanted to have this party, I guess. It means so much to me that you guys are here. I don't know how I would have handled it without you, Sam." I looked up to see Julie standing in the doorway.

"I didn't realize everyone would be here already," Julie said. "Hey, Sam, you look awesome, same as always. I can't believe you have twins."

"Hey, Julie," Sam chirped, jumping off the bed to give Julie a hug. "I'll leave you two alone for a while to catch up. It's great to see you again, Julie. I hear your girls are adorable. Oh, and Jenn, everybody is out on errands for the party—Henry, the kids, Jacob and Betsy—so are you OK here?"

"Sure, I'm fine," I answered.

"I'll watch over her," Julie said. She seemed strangely upbeat, as if buoyed by good news she couldn't wait to tell. I knew her moods as well as my own. She was smartly dressed in a brown turtleneck, skirt, and flat boots—very crisp and equestrian, I thought.

"I guess home really does agree with you, Jennifer," She said, bending to kiss my cheek. "You look 100 percent better since the last time I saw you. I really mean it. Now, what about you and… Henry?" she asked, coyly.

The last time she saw me, it was Alex and me. Good ol' Julie, going for the jugular, as always. My face flushed as I focused on the wall just beyond her left shoulder. We were locked in a life-long rivalry that wouldn't ever be over. It shaped our relationship as sisters, both in childhood and in adulthood. Any peace between us would be uneasy, at best, but would be built upon what was left unsaid, rather than what was spoken. We both knew how to pick the words that stabbed each other to the core. Always had, always would, but suddenly I needed Julie to know I was simply tired of fighting. "Julie, whatever you think of me, whatever you think happened with Alex, there are two sides to every story. I wish you could be on my side, because you are my sister, my only sister, and I do love you," I said.

"What do you mean? You've used poor Alex for decades—can't you see that? And finally, when he was free of you and maybe finding happiness with me, you lure him back in!" she yelled. "How is that being on *my* side?"

"What? You've got to be kidding. Julie, look at me. Look at me. I have cancer; I'm sick. I'm in a hospital bed. I'm not alluring or luring. You've got this all wrong," I said, standing up now, looking her in the eye. And then things got worse.

Behind her my door opened, and Alex walked in.

"Oh my god," I stammered before finding my way back to the throne.

"Ladies," Alex said, looking first at Julie and then at me. "I hate to be the cause of such consternation, not when we were all getting along so well. Jenn and me, Julie and me. Who wants a kiss to feel better?"

Julie backed up until she was between Alex and me, shielding me with her petite frame. "Alex, you aren't welcome here—get out now," she said. Her voice quivered, but she was calm.

I kept my eyes focused on Alex—on his crazy brown eyes; the same evil I saw at the lake house shined back. Slowly, I moved my left hand toward my cell phone on the bedside table.

"Jenn, you look lovely as usual. And, Julie, my number two, you should know better than to threaten me. You know I'm a bit explosive—just look at the bruises on your sister," Alex said.

I grabbed my phone and punched 9-1—when Alex wrenched it out of my hand. "No need to call anyone, dear, I'll be leaving in a moment. Just wanted to tell both of you good-bye and good riddance. I'm going back home. So sorry I'll miss your party."

Julie pushed him away from me and moved between us. "Alex, leave her alone!" she screamed.

His eyes flashed, and I knew he would hurt Julie too. "Run, Julie! My god, Alex, stop!"

Suddenly, Henry was there. He was on top of Alex, and they were rolling around on the floor. I heard Julie yelling into her telephone, saying it was an emergency as she ran to the doorway where Hank and Hannah, who had arrived home with Henry to this chaos, stood.

I watched as Henry, a college boxer, landed a blow to Alex's nose, seeming to flatten his entire face. And Alex stopped moving.

"Henry, stop this minute!" Julie yelled from the hall. "The kids!"

"Dada," Hank cried.

Henry stopped punching and lifted Alex up by his shirt collar, holding his bloodied face close to his own. "If you ever come near any of my family again, I will kill you," he whispered, loud enough for only the three of us in my room to hear. Henry marched him out of my room—and finally, out of our lives.

Julie brought the kids in, and the four of us cuddled on the throne until Henry called for Julie. "The police need to speak with you," he said.

She squeezed my hand. "I'll be right back," she said to me.

"Mama, what happen?" Hank asked finally, when he stopped crying. "Why Dada hurt man?"

"Daddy hurt the bad man to protect Mommy and Aunt Julie. Daddy is a hero," I told him. He nodded and burrowed under the covers.

Julie and Henry came back to my room together, Henry with a huge bandage and ice on his right hand.

"Out of practice," he said simply before giving me a big kiss on the lips.

"You were amazing," I said. "I am so glad you came back when you did."

"Me too," Henry answered and scooped up Hank and Hannah, not an easy feat with an injured fist. "I'll put them down for their naps, and I'll be back. Julie, watch over her for me."

"That did a lot of good last time," Julie said. She perched on the throne next to me and dropped her head. When she looked back at me, she was transformed, tears running down her face. "He conned me. He used me to get to you. All the time he was trying to get information about you. I slept with him, Jenn. I thought he loved me, that we would be together. I never imagined you would leave with him, that you still liked him. What have I done?"

"It's OK, Julie, it is," I said, sitting up next to my sister on the bed. "I wanted to believe in him, that he was my friend. He tricked me too. But it's over now."

"I'm so sorry Jenn," Julie said.

"I'm sorry too, Julie."

We sat side by side, quietly on my bed, as peaceful as we'd been in ages.

When Henry came back to join us, Julie stood to leave but leaned toward me once again. Reaching for my hand, she looked me straight in the eyes and kissed me gently on the forehead. "Good-bye for now—*not* forever, Jennifer. Enjoy your party." At the door, she half-turned and waved, mouthing a silent "love you" before leaving me to wonder if sibling rivalry was just part of loving, confirming who you are at heart.

18

Warning: Individual results may vary.

WHEN HENRY WOKE ME, I REALIZED I'D HAD A SURPRISINGLY restful night's sleep, considering.

"It's not too late to cancel. I mean, they can come in, grab some food, and leave. You don't have to see anybody," Henry said. His eyes sparkled their bright, brilliant blue as he looked at me. "Honey, I would cry too, if it happened to me. What you've been through. Anybody would cry. So really, take it easy on yourself. You only need to do what you want to do."

Lying down next to me on our double-wide, hospital-utility but fine-hotel bed, he started to kiss my neck. "Do you want to do this?" he asked.

"Oh yes," I said, but then I pushed him away. "I want to do that for the rest of our lives—but today, we're having a party. Now, help me get ready, you sex-starved husband, you." We both laughed as he stood up and held out his hand to help me. "How's your hand?" I asked, rubbing the knuckles he used to break Alex's nose.

"I'm fine," he beamed. "I can still protect my girl."

"He's just lucky you didn't kill him," I said.

"I could have, except the kids were watching," Henry said. "Enough about him. Let's focus on today. I'm really worried seeing all of these people will, well, make me lose you again. To the depression, to the despondency, to somebody else."

"Don't be ridiculous. We'll never lose each other again," I said. "I don't want to cry anymore. I want to be happy. I'm ready to celebrate the good. I'm getting stronger every day. I promise. Meg's still coming, right?" I asked. Meg was our wedding photographer, new-baby photographer, and my inspiration for wanting to get serious about photography someday. "I'm not using the wheelchair. I'll stay in here, and you guys can send people in, OK?"

"Of course, honey," Henry said, wiping the worry from his face and steeling himself for the day. For me. "As you wish. The caterers will be here by 9:00 a.m."

"Thank you, love of my life," I said to Henry, before he bowed. After all we'd been through, the past year, month, day, even, with an uncertain future, I wanted my moments to count. I was smoothing things over with my sister, and I wanted to have loving moments with Henry. I wanted to prove to him that I could have other people in my life again, that I could be multidimensional without being a cheater. I needed to get back to normal again, to the place where I was working, running a business in the real world, raising two amazing kids. A place where I was trustworthy, faithful, and in love. And we would. We would get there, together, and I would prove to him it was possible through these parties. He'd learn more about me. And these visits, these memories, could end up being all he had left, for the kids, for him.

"How about bringing Hank and Hannah in for a visit? That would be great," I suggested just before he walked out the door.

The lines around Henry's mouth relaxed, and his eyes took on a bit of a twinkle. He wanted connection too. He wanted it to be OK. Our two kids were us, our family. And the four of us together would bring me back to our life.

"The kids are really excited," he said. "I'll have Paige bring them in after they're ready. And honey," Henry added with a smile, "why don't you start getting ready?"

"Yes, sir," I said, saluting. The house's previous owners had a wheelchair-bound relative living with them, and they had added for her use a full bath completely wheelchair accessible. We'd joked before about having his mom or my mother live with us at some point. We didn't know it would become perfect for me at age thirty-four.

Like many big events, including my wedding reception, the party was over too soon. A few words here, a few words there. Even though the guests were supposed to sign in, smile for a photo, and come in to see me one by one, they ended up arriving in clumps, as if in a unit bigger than one they could handle the reality of what they might encounter. The longer it had been since I'd seen one visitor, the bigger the clump surrounding that person grew.

My favorite elementary school teacher brought her entire family. They huddled around the throne, listening as she and I exchanged remembrances. And it was great seeing former neighbors, several old bosses, and even favorite professors, who arrived together and visited in a clump of four. It wasn't the privacy I had planned but it was still better than waiting until my funeral.

Ralph's wife, Barb, surprised me, walking into my room by herself, her elegant grace wrapped around her like a cloak.

"I wanted you to have something to remember Ralph by," she said, handing me a wrapped package.

"I don't need anything to remind me of Ralph. He'll live in my heart forever," I said, tears springing to my eyes as I opened the gift. It was a photo of Ralph and me playing Scrabble. "I'll treasure this forever, Barb. Thank you."

We held each other tight before she broke the embrace. "Keep getting better, Jenn. Ralph knew you would make it. Live a full life for him too," she added, and she was gone.

Daddy was outside the door, holding court, coordinating traffic flow, quite the Grandville celebrity, the burger king.

"That's my girl in there. Don't worry, she'll beat this," he boasted. "Hell, she's twenty thousand times better than she was just yesterday. Before long, she'll be on a buying trip with Jacob and bossing us all around, like always."

Daddy. We may not have had the perfect family, but he was still an extraordinary parent, doing the best he could for me. Believing in me no matter what. Hearing his strong voice outside my door all day kept me grounded. He was the beginning and the end of my receiving line. Every twenty minutes or so, he'd pop in to check on me. Touching my head, asking if I needed anything. We'd come to a certain peace between us, a truce. We were back in balance again too. I cherished the comfort of a booming voice just outside my door.

Was any family perfect, really? A family is made up of individuals, each with baggage, issues. At their best, they build each other up. At their worst, they let each other down. I'd been blessed: both my parents were alive—and somewhat available. A privileged upbringing paid for by my daddy's single-minded pursuit of success and my mother's sacrifices. That they grew and changed along the way was normal, expected. I guess I always more or less accepted Daddy's priority of work over family, but I could never imagine putting my kids second to anything or anyone, no matter what. Not for lust, not for business, not for a second chance at love.

But that's what I almost did with Alex, I realized. Without thinking of anyone but myself, I'd almost had an affair just to feel less lonely. I shuddered and tried to put a smile on my face before the next group was ushered in.

Henry, Betsy, and Jacob played the perfect hosts. Bringing groups in and out. Making sure people didn't take up too much time. Listening for the signal over the baby monitor when I'd had enough of one particular visitor or another.

It was better than our wedding reception in some ways. Back then, nobody was on the other end of a baby monitor to come to my rescue. And one of my bridesmaids' husbands—no one ever came clean—made it his mission to get Henry drunk. I, on the other hand, had been the epitome of the princess bride—no drinks, no man, just a big white dress and a lot of lipstick smears on my cheeks. When I finally found Henry, slurring and attempting the Russian polka, I knew our first night as a married couple was going to be less than stellar.

But as always, when I needed somebody, my friends were there. After Henry passed out in our honeymoon suite at the hotel, I joined the rest of the wedding party already in progress at a bar down the street from the hotel. Friends, to me, were, are, and always would provide the meaning and core of my life. Henry knew it. That's why I loved him.

And so the day went. Some of my visitors brought photos of us together, reminding me, among other insights, that perms were never my friend. Ever. Others brought cards for me to read later. Nancy, who lived across the street, brought me a huge plate of cookies. She said she couldn't help herself. Whenever she went to somebody's house—for anything—she brought cookies. I appreciated the gesture, hers and everybody's. This wasn't easy.

I guess when I dreamed up this event as a close to my life, I never thought it would happen. Sure, I'd planned for it, thought about it, even fought for my right to have it, and the very process had given me another reason to struggle through each day. But once the party started, I sort of felt like an untouchable item in a white dress again—the center of attention but not part of the festivities.

This time, though, I wasn't in all white, standing on the brink of a promising future. I was in an oversized hospital bed, with Mother's artful makeup and a bright smile painted on my face as I tried to reach out to people who had touched my life in ways great and small. Many guests entered my room talking gaily among themselves but fell awkwardly silent as they approached me on my throne. For some, it was their first visit since my diagnosis, and their guilt was palpable as they touched my hand or whispered a greeting. I didn't want anyone to feel guilty, I just wanted them to know they were important in my life and a part of who I was, and I tried to convey my feelings to the braver of the guests. Some visits were as superficial as an afternoon tea, but in the end, I decided that was OK too. The me I was to most of them was a person in their past. The current Jennifer was as foreign to them as she was to me.

A couple of my teachers walked in, ending self-reflection for a moment. Both had saved some of my work and used it as examples for their current classes. They brought along copies to remind me of my efforts. That was nice, to know I could possibly be an inspiration. Of course, no former math teachers arrived with efforts to brag about. But I didn't expect that much.

Periodically, Henry would take up position on the end of the throne, a protective conversation starter and my guardian angel, ready to shoo folks out of the room if I gave him a hint. As he sat watching me interact with my former teachers, I saw a tear slide down his cheek, a tear he quickly brushed away before he thought I would notice it. *Oh Henry, everything will be all right.* Before Henry ushered them out, he gave me a kiss on the cheek.

As they left, I realized that, no matter how many people you fill your life with—or in my case, your good-bye party with—everyone's journey is singular. We are, no matter how well-adjusted, no matter how happily partnered, and no matter how loved by others, alone.

A large clump of the Loop's best customers arrived then, all together—about the size of a country club tennis team. Henry followed them in, dividing the women into two social clusters, taking half back out and leaving the other half in my room to coo and cluck at me. What did they represent to me? I tried to figure that out while they were chatting at me, with each other. A business success? Obviously, since they validated my taste and my concept for a store. A connection to my mother as I viewed her from my childhood, merrily playing tennis, shopping, and lunching? Probably. But again, that longing for a connection, for understanding, was in the end elusive. These women didn't have a real connection to me, just to my clothes, my sense of style. But that was OK. That's how it was supposed to be among us, right?

But why was I so glad, very glad, they were there? I guess, down deep, these women represented some of what I wanted in life, not just as customers in my store. They were clear in their expectations. They were beautiful. Privileged. Spoiled. Pampered. Outwardly, they were the envy of society. Connected. Dressed by me in the epitome of you've-made-it clothing.

On the flip side, they represented to me the vulnerability associated with that precarious life. Of looking good, of living well, but not of having an exit plan or a backup. Financially, if their husbands left—died, found a younger woman, got a gambling addiction, whatever—their lives were toast. Gone. With a few wealthy exceptions. That fear I kept to myself. Why worry for them if they weren't worried?

Style, fashion, that's what brought us together and bonded us, not impending doom. For the moment. At the store. With Jacob. With me. At the Loop, we all cared about what it meant to be current, the feeling you got when what you were wearing felt right, when what other people said as you walked down the street made you walk taller, when the right clothes made you feel confident inside. Like nothing or nobody else could do for you, sometimes. That shopping urge. It was really an identity urge.

I created the place where they could come. From tennis. From a bad morning with the kids. After a fight with an overcontrolling husband. When life wasn't working out, however it wasn't working out, the Loop was where you went to find other women who felt the same.

And that was my place. Their place. The Loop. That these women selected, appreciated, purchased items I'd gone to market for—I guess it was more important to me than I knew. More central than I'd admitted. They validated my career-woman self, while piling guilt—not intentionally, on most days—on that same working-mom self. Sharing a sense of style and judging—quietly—each other's choices. Wasn't that our way? As women?

Is that what happened to me? Did my sense of self collapse when I couldn't hide behind the façade of my perfect house, perfect clothes, perfect marriage, and perfect career? With the cancer diagnosis, time stopped. Everything that mattered before suddenly didn't. All that mattered was surviving. Surviving for my children, if I was honest. They were the first and only priority beyond beating this invasion.

I had started to see Henry as a soldier in the fight, helping me along, of course, but with primary duties of preserving and protecting the kids for when I returned. I didn't see him as a partner or a lover once this happened. How could I have expected him to see me as a lover with all my body had been through? When none of the beautiful clothes fit, when my hair was gone, when the scars oozed. And if I couldn't accept myself, how I looked, I think I may have subconsciously tried to make it easier on Henry by blocking him out, by becoming his platonic friend, his general directing orders from the throne.

That's what I'd done, to me, to us. It was much more than dreaming of the past, or escaping with Alex. I'd left him emotionally long before the confines of Shady Valley forced me to leave him physically.

But he'd stayed. Even as my confidence in myself left, Henry stayed. Even when I ran away with Alex, Henry stayed. This realization sent shivers down my spine. I needed to see Henry, alone. Now.

Ann, one of my favorites of the group, was speaking. I'd clearly tuned out. I smiled, hoping she hadn't noticed the lapse. "And when you helped my daughter find the prom dress, it made her feel so special and really just made her night, a really important night, special, because she knew she looked good. I just know you'll get better. We all need you—you help to make us look good and feel good; that and, well, we miss you." Ann finished with a cough.

Even though I'd missed most of her speech, her point was clear. And I loved her for it. As I smiled up at her, she dabbed at tears.

"Thanks, Ann. Thanks to all of you for coming today. Really, you don't know how much it means, has meant, to me that you support the store. And you understand me. That you like what I like…Could you send Henry in, please?"

Nodding, Ann took the lead as they each, one by one, kissed me on the cheek or the forehead or squeezed my hand and hustled out. All the while, I felt more connected to them, each one, than I ever had before. I didn't know if they felt the same. Perhaps they had known we were the same all along.

"Honey, I heard you ask for me over the monitor," Henry said, bursting into the room, thankfully alone. "Is everything all right?"

I reached over and turned off the monitor. "I just wanted you to know how much I love you," I said, dabbing at the tears as Mother had showed me how to do to keep my mascara intact. I still had quite a few party groups to see. "You stayed with me through all of this. You could have left. You could have—"

"No, Jennifer, I couldn't have done anything other than this," Henry said, sitting next to me on the throne. "I don't want to be anywhere but here with you, forever. In sickness and in health, you're the love of my life for as long as you'll have me."

We sat hugging on the bed until Daddy knocked on the door. "Hey, Jennifer, there are a bunch of folks waiting to see you, so if you could tell your husband to get on out of there, we'll get this party going."

Henry smiled, stood up, and straightened the covers around me. "Just a little more party to go until it's you and me," he said. He turned the monitor back on and gave me the thumbs-up as he left the room.

The rest of the day, I enjoyed listening to the ebb and flow of people in our home. Of shared joy at long-misplaced friends, the crescendo of a final farewell. Sure, there were plenty of tears but plenty of laughter too. All in all, I was enjoying this much more than I would my funeral service, I was sure of that.

Mother had arrived before the party, as promised, and we shared a few quiet moments as she clucked and fussed over my hair and makeup. Although I redid my hair as soon as she left the room, I appreciated the attention. She popped in sporadically during the day to "freshen me up," as she called it. It was her way of showing love, I realized. You look good, you feel good, she always said, not realizing the irony, I supposed, of my particular situation.

When Katie and Maddie came in for their official visit, it was awkward. As we were planning the party, it had somehow seemed fine. But now that the party was over, we were all speechless. Maybe I'd talked too much anyway. Maybe I'd placed too much emphasis on the party and not enough on time with my friends here, now.

"Well, Jennifer, it's not like we won't see you or anything. Book club's in two weeks. Have you started *Red Badge of Courage* yet?" Katie asked, her hair a perfect blond helmet, her skin tanned from her trip to Cabo.

"Nope. Sorry," I laughed. "This will be the week. I promise. I start my new treatment on Monday, and I have nothing but time on my hands." The statement hung in the air, heavy with meaning.

"Great," Maddie's voice cracked. "Well, I'd better run. I need a smoke, and you need your rest. See you soon, Jenn."

"Me too," Katie said, tears welling in her eyes.

"Guys, please, stop being awkward. I'll see you in a couple weeks, OK? Thanks for everything."

Jacob walked in and saved us from degenerating into a real breakdown. Katie and Maddie hugged me quickly and each gave Jacob a quick hug as they left the room.

"Well, gorgeous. What did you think? Did you have a fun party?" he asked.

"It was perfect—what did you think? And why haven't you brought up the Alex incident?" I asked.

"Oh, honey, yesterday? That's old news," Jacob said. "Henry saved the day, knocking out the crazy old boyfriend and protecting you and your scheming sister. Alex posted bail, and I bet he runs away to Texas or wherever he can crawl in a hole. Do I have that right?" he asked.

"I think you've got it all," I laughed.

"As for the party, the chilled shrimp should've been deveined, but besides that, exquisite," Jacob said. "Lots of cute guys, if you like preppy, but don't tell Nelson I noticed."

"Who? My friends?" I asked, thinking most were looking fairly middle-aged and boring.

"No, of course not. No offense, but they were all old. I'm talking about the waiters," he said.

"Jacob," I said as he bent down and gave me a hug. "Stop it. No tears. I'll talk to you tomorrow, you goofball. The party's over, that's all. Everything else is the same."

"Are you sure, Jennifer? Because I want it to be. I want you to get better, more than I can ever say, and I love you more than you know," he said, tears trickling down his cheeks.

"I know. And I love you, too. So knock it off. I don't want to cry anymore right now," I said, pushing him up, out of our hug.

"Call me tomorrow?" he asked, extracting a tissue and blowing his nose.

"Count on it. You better go spend some time with Nelson. He made quite a sacrifice by working the store for us today," I said.

"Yeah. I know. He said to tell you he would've been here, except he had to make money for you. Bye."

As my eyelids began to close, I realized someone had walked into the room when Jacob left. Daddy. I smiled up at him through the sog of tears as he pulled a chair next to the throne. He looked tired from his daylong efforts as doorman-greeter. Puffy, black circles ringed the bottoms of each eye. His gray hair was thinning at the top, I noticed suddenly. Daddy was getting old.

"I hope the party wasn't too hard on you, sweetheart," he said, holding my hand. "I know how important it was for you to see everyone. It did this old heart good, I can tell you that. A lot of memories. You're a very special woman, and I love you."

"Don't cry, Daddy," I said, crying. "I love you too, so much. I am so glad you were here today. Thank you for helping."

"All I want is for you to get well, that's it. I'd do anything, you know that," he said.

"Yes, I do, I do know that," I answered as exhaustion overwhelmed me, and I fell asleep holding Daddy's hand.

19

Warning: Use only as directed.

IT WAS ALREADY NOON. I HADN'T SLEPT IN SO LATE SINCE MY COL-lege days. I guessed the party took more of a toll than I realized. Many of my out-of-town guests were gone, and any who stayed were visiting other friends or touring old haunts. On Monday we would begin the next miracle trial drug. Maybe. I wasn't sure if I was up to it. Maybe I'd already used up my miracles, living as long as I had. Maybe it was time to let go. Go peacefully.

"Jennifer?" Sam said from the doorway. She was an out-of-towner who lingered. She was dressed in jeans and a white blouse. She looked like she could walk onto any college campus and fit in with the undergrads.

"I'm awake," I said. "Come on in, Sam. Sorry I conked out on you guys for so long. I know it's time for you to head back to your life too, right?"

"I wish so much I didn't have to," Sam said. "I'm sorry."

"No tears, please—the doctors are trying to rehydrate me," I said, tears welling up in my eyes too. "You'll never know how much it meant having you here. Helping me with my party. Spending time with me. It's been so wonderful."

"Yeah, like an extended slumber party. I called Mike, just to see if he could handle the kids and the house and getting ready for back to school just a little longer, but he needs me. You know how helpless men are. But I'm coming back just as soon as I can."

"I'll email you copies of Meg's photos," I said. "Thank you, for being here."

"You're an inspiration, Jennifer. Keep strong. I think this new treatment will do it. You'll be in our prayers," Sam said, giving me a big hug. "I love you."

"I love you too," I said.

"Doctor's orders, no crying," Betsy said as she joined us.

"Oh good, Betsy, I'm glad you're here. I didn't want to leave her sad." Sam sniffed.

"I'm OK. You go on so you don't miss your flight. Go. I'm fine," I lied, and she did leave, stopping on the walkway and bending and waving to me through the window. Knowing I could see her, even if she couldn't see me.

"Boy, you've got great friends," Betsy said, plunking down on the throne.

"I know. I'm so lucky. And the best one is sitting right here with me now," I said.

"Well, I certainly take the prize for longest—mind you, I didn't say oldest." Betsy teased. "Honey, you don't look so good."

"Maybe I should just sleep a little more," I answered.

"That's a good idea. I'll have Paige bring the kids in quickly and then take them up for their naps. Henry can stay and tuck you in," Betsy said.

"That would be nice if you could do that, Betsy," I said. "I was thinking, if it's a girl?"

"Of course, her name is Jennifer. With all this morning sickness I'm having, I think it must be a girl. I didn't have any with Zach. Jennifer's a feisty fetus already," she said with a smile. "Sleep well. I love you."

As Betsy headed for the door, I called after her, "You too, Betsy. Forever."

"Honey?" Henry said softly, his shape replacing Betsy's in the doorway.

"I'm not asleep. Just resting," I said, smiling up at Hannah in his arms as Hank barreled through the door.

"Night-night, Mommy. I'm taking a nap too," Hank said, climbing up on the throne and tossing his arms around my neck.

"Have a good nap, my little man. Who loves you to the moon and back?" I asked.

"You do. And I love you to the sun and the stars and back," he said. Henry placed a very tired Hannah next to me on the bed. The baby-powder smell of her body and softness of her skin comforted me as I hugged her close.

"Bobble, Momma?" Hannah asked.

"Paige has your bottle for you, baby. I just need a good hug," I said, squeezing her tight. "Have a great nap, my princess. I love you."

Paige came and scooped up each child and took my angels to their naps. Hank waved as he disappeared through the door.

Henry sat beside me on the bed, a look of concern on his face. "I'm worried that yesterday was too much for you. I want you to keep resting, and know I love you. I was proud of how wonderful you were with…with everyone yesterday. I think it was special. Just like you wanted. I just hope—" His voice broke, and I realized he was crying.

"Why crying?" I asked. My lips didn't seem to want to make all the words I was thinking, just every couple of words. I hadn't known I could be so deeply tired. I wanted to sink back into my cushion of sleep, to be enveloped by it entirely.

"I want you to know how happy you've made me in my life. I am here, always and forever for you. You know how much you mean to Hank and Hannah. They love you so much, honey, and they always will."

I know that, I thought but couldn't speak. Even though I knew Henry wasn't quite ready for it, I fall asleep.

Have you ever considered what would have happened in your life if you had married someone different, especially if you had a first love? Do you have someone who "got away"?

Although Jennifer's situation is bleak, she finds much to be hopeful for and keeps herself busy planning a party. While that may not be your choice of activities if you were in her situation, was it a valuable pursuit for her in the end?

Jennifer and Ralph have a special relationship. How would you describe their friendship, and why is Ralph such an important character in the story?

The author chose gravely ill cancer patients to be the protagonists of the story. Is cancer the antagonist, or is it something else?

What do you think of Alex? How is he similar to and different from Henry?

What relevance do Jacob and Clothes the Loop have to the story?

Do you believe Jennifer falls asleep at the end of the story, or do you believe she dies? What does your answer say about you and your outlook on life, if anything?

ACKNOWLEDGMENTS

THANK YOU FOR READING THIS BOOK. CANCER HAS TOUCHED almost all of us, some lightly and some, like the fictional characters in this book and too many of my friends and family, with a knockout punch. The disease and its treatments are handled fictitiously in this novel. However, Jennifer's grace is emblematic of many young mothers who have faced the same dastardly opponent, often with triumph.

Thank you to my agent, Amanda Luedeke, who believes in this story and the future.

Thank you to my friends and early readers—especially Elizabeth Paulsen, Colleen Sturdivant, and Melissa Cavanaugh—who have trudged through more versions of this novel than I ever thought possible to write over the many years it has taken this story to come to life.

Thank you to Laura Meehan, Kristin Thiel, and the team at Indigo for making sure my words make sense and to Erin Corrigan for amazing cover art.

A warm hug and thank you to the amazing and supportive women's fiction writers I have had the pleasure of getting to know both in person and online during the last few years. This career wouldn't be the same without you and your support. A special thanks to Jenna Blum, Barbara DeMarco-Barrett, Lian Dolan, Tracey Garvis Graves, Amy Hatvany, Katrina Kittle, Jane Porter, Anita Hughes, Suzanne Redfearn, and the entire staff of Laguna Beach Books.

To my family, which now includes three dogs and a fish, for your support and unbridled excitement whenever I need it most. I love you all.

If you enjoyed *In the Mirror*, consider these other novels by Kaira Rouda:

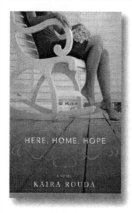

Here, Home, Hope
The absorbing witty story of one mother's journey from midlife crisis to reinvention.

Kelly Johnson is a 39-year-old wife and mother stuck in the rut of her suburban life. With hilarity, endearing gusto, and charm, Kelly dives into new projects armed with Post-It notes, revisiting old memories and rediscovering passions. As her midlife crisis comes crashing down, Kelly ultimately grows into a woman empowered by her own reinvention.

"Reading Kaira Rouda is like getting together with one of your best friends – fun, fast and full of great advice!"
- Claire Cook, bestselling author of *Must Love Dogs*

All the Difference
The suspenseful story of three women whose lives become entangled by their choices and how, ultimately, one turns to murder to achieve her goals.

Beautiful Ellen abandons her life as a successful fund-raiser for that of an isolated housewife for her husband, whose affairs become increasingly hard to ignore. Television anchor Laura is driven to succeed, and move to a major media market, whatever the cost. Angie is a luckless waitress waiting for Mr. Right to save her from a life spent making bad choices, particularly when it comes to men.

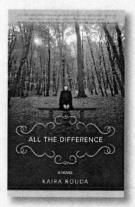

"A murder mystery that kept me guessing until the end, with lovable characters who made me laugh and cry. Kaira Rouda has done it again."
- *USA Today* bestselling author Melissa Foster

And coming soon, *LINES IN THE SAND*...

CPSIA information can be obtained at www.ICGtesting.com
Printed in the USA
LVOW13s2118300414

383887LV00008BA/1033/P